Burn Resuscitation

Editors

KEVIN N. FOSTER
DANIEL M. CARUSO

CRITICAL CARE CLINICS

www.criticalcare.theclinics.com

Consulting Editor
RICHARD W. CARLSON

October 2016 • Volume 32 • Number 4

ELSEVIER

1600 John F. Kennedy Boulevard • Suite 1800 • Philadelphia, Pennsylvania, 19103-2899

http://www.theclinics.com

CRITICAL CARE CLINICS Volume 32, Number 4
October 2016 ISSN 0749-0704, ISBN-13: 978-0-323-46304-1

Editor: Patrick Manley
Developmental Editor: Casey Jackson

Critical Care Clinics (ISSN: 0749-0704) is published quarterly by Elsevier Inc., 360 Park Avenue South, New York, NY 10010-1710. Months of issue are January, April, July, and October. Business and Editorial Offices: 1600 John F. Kennedy Blvd., Suite 1800, Philadelphia, PA 19103-2899. Customer Service Office: 6277 Sea Harbor Drive, Orlando, FL 32887-4800. Periodicals postage paid at New York, NY and additional mailing offices. Subscription prices are $215.00 per year for US individuals, $551.00 per year for US institution, $100.00 per year for US students and residents, $255.00 per year for Canadian individuals, $691.00 per year for Canadian institutions, $300.00 per year for international individuals, $691.00 per year for international institutions and $150.00 per year for Canadian and foreign students/residents. To receive student/resident rate, orders must be accompanied by name of affiliated institution, date of term, and the signature of program/residency coordinator on institution letterhead. Orders will be billed at individual rate until proof of status is received. Foreign air speed delivery is included in all *Clinics* subscription prices. All prices are subject to change without notice. POSTMASTER: Send address changes to *Critical Care Clinics*, Elsevier Periodicals Customer Service, 11830 Westline Industrial Drive, St. Louis, MO 63146. **Customer Service: 1-800-654-2452 (US). From outside of the US, call 1-314-447-8871. Fax: 1-314-447-8029. E-mail: journalscustomerservice-usa@elsevier.com (for print support) or journalsonlinesupport-usa@elsevier.com (for online support).**

Reprints. For copies of 100 or more of articles in this publication, please contact the Commercial Reprints Department, Elsevier Inc., 360 Park Avenue South, New York, NY 10010-1710. Tel.: 212-633-3874; Fax: 212-633-3820; E-mail: reprints@elsevier.com.

Critical Care Clinics is also published in Spanish by Editorial Inter-Medica, Junin 917, 1er A, 1113, Buenos Aires, Argentina.

Critical Care Clinics is covered in *MEDLINE/PubMed (Index Medicus), EMBASE/Excerpta Medica, Current Concepts/Clinical Medicine, ISI/BIOMED, and Chemical Abstracts.*

Contributors

CONSULTING EDITOR

RICHARD W. CARLSON, MD, PhD, MCCM, MACP
Chairman Emeritus, Department of Medicine, Maricopa Medical Center, Phoenix, Arizona;
Professor, Mayo Clinic College of Medicine, Scottsdale, Arizona; Professor, University of
Arizona College of Medicine, Phoenix, Arizona

EDITORS

KEVIN N. FOSTER, MD, MBA, FACS
Director of Burn Services, The Arizona Burn Center, Professor, University of Arizona
College of Medicine, Phoenix, Arizona

DANIEL M. CARUSO, MD, FACS
Professor and Executive Chair, Department of Surgery, University of Arizona College of
Medicine; The Arizona Burn Center, Maricopa Medical Center, Phoenix, Arizona

AUTHORS

BRETT D. ARNOLDO, MD
Division of Burns, Trauma, and Critical Care, Department of Surgery, University of
Texas–Southwestern Medical Center, Dallas, Texas

ELISHA G. BROWNSON, MD
Department of Surgery, Harborview Medical Center, Seattle, Washington

LEOPOLDO C. CANCIO, MD, FACS, FCCM
Clinical Professor of Surgery, US Army Institute of Surgical Research, JBSA Fort Sam
Houston, Texas

ROBERT CARTOTTO, MD, FRCS(C)
Department of Surgery, Ross Tilley Burn Centre, Sunnybrook Health Sciences Centre,
University of Toronto, Toronto, Ontario, Canada

DANIEL M. CARUSO, MD, FACS
Professor and Executive Chair, Department of Surgery, University of Arizona College of
Medicine; The Arizona Burn Center, Maricopa Medical Center, Phoenix, Arizona

KEVIN K. CHUNG, MD
United States Army Institute of Surgical Research, JBSA Fort Sam Houston, Texas;
Department of Surgery, Uniformed Services University of the Health Sciences, Bethesda,
Maryland

IAN R. DRISCOLL, MD
United States Army Institute of Surgical Research, JBSA Fort Sam Houston, Texas; Department of Surgery, Uniformed Services University of the Health Sciences, Bethesda, Maryland

PHILIP FIDLER, MD, FACS
Medical Director, Swedish Hospital, Englewood, Colorado

KEVIN N. FOSTER, MD, MBA, FACS
Director of Burn Services, The Arizona Burn Center, Professor, University of Arizona College of Medicine, Phoenix, Arizona

BRUCE C. FRIEDMAN, MD
JM Still Burn Center at Doctor's Hospital, Augusta, Georgia

NICOLE GIBRAN, MD, FACS
Medical Director, UW Burn Center, Seattle, Washington

DAVID GREENHALGH, MD, FACS
Department of Surgery, Shriners Hospitals for Children Northern California, University of California, Davis, Sacramento, California

DAVID T. HARRINGTON, MD, FACS
Director, Rhode Island Burn Center, Rhode Island Hospital; Professor of Surgery, Warren Alpert Medical School of Brown University, Providence, Rhode Island

ERICA I. HODGMAN, MD
Division of Burns, Trauma, and Critical Care, Department of Surgery, University of Texas–Southwestern Medical Center, Dallas, Texas

JAMES JENG, MD, FACS
Associate Professor of Surgery, Mount Sinai Healthcare System, New York, New York

GEORGE C. KRAMER, PhD
Director, Resuscitation Research Laboratory, Department of Anesthesiology, University of Texas Medical Branch at Galveston, Galveston, Texas

MARC R. MATTHEWS, MD, FACS
Associate Professor, Department of Surgery, University of Arizona College of Medicine; The Arizona Burn Center, Maricopa Medical Center, Phoenix, Arizona

AMR MOGHAZY, MD, MSc, PhD
Associate Professor of Plastic Surgery and Burns Faculty of Medicine, Suez Canal University; Consultant of Plastic Surgery and Burns, Suez Canal University Hospitals, Ismailia, Egypt

TINA L. PALMIERI, MD, FACS, FCCM
Professor, Shriners Hospitals for Children Northern California, University of California Davis, Sacramento, California

MICHAEL PECK, MD, ScD
Department of Surgery, Arizona Burn Center, Maricopa Medical Center, Phoenix, Arizona

TAM N. PHAM, MD
Department of Surgery, Harborview Medical Center, Seattle, Washington

HERB A. PHELAN, MD
Division of Burns, Trauma, and Critical Care, Department of Surgery, University of Texas–Southwestern Medical Center, Dallas, Texas

LISA RAE, MD
Assistant Professor of Surgery, Departments of Trauma, Surgical Critical Care and Emergency General Surgery, Vanderbilt University Medical Center, Nashville, Tennessee

JULIE A. RIZZO, MD
United States Army Institute of Surgical Research, JBSA Fort Sam Houston, Texas; Department of Surgery, Uniformed Services University of the Health Sciences, Bethesda, Maryland

MATTHEW P. ROWAN, PhD
United States Army Institute of Surgical Research, JBSA Fort Sam Houston, Texas

JEFFREY R. SAFFLE, MD, FACS
Professor Emeritus, University of Utah Health Center, Lake Elmo, Minnesota

JOSE SALINAS, PhD
Task Area Manager, Comprehensive Intensive Care Research, US Army Institute of Surgical Research, JBSA Fort Sam Houston, Texas

MADHU SUBRAMANIAN, MD
Division of Burns, Trauma, and Critical Care, Department of Surgery, University of Texas–Southwestern Medical Center, Dallas, Texas

STEVEN E. WOLF, MD
Division of Burns, Trauma, and Critical Care, Department of Surgery, University of Texas–Southwestern Medical Center, Dallas, Texas

Contents

Burn trauma in the current age of medical care still portends a 3% to 8% mortality. Of patients who die from their burn injuries, 58% of deaths occur in the first 72 hours after injury, indicating death from the initial burn shock is still a major cause of burn mortality. Significant thermal injury incites an inflammatory response, which distinguishes burns from other trauma. This article focuses on the current understanding of the pathophysiology of burn shock, the inflammatory response, and the direction of research and targeted therapies to improve resuscitation, morbidity, and mortality.

Colloids have been used in varying capacities throughout the history of formula-based burn resuscitation. There is sound experimental evidence that demonstrates colloids' ability to improve intravascular colloid osmotic pressure, expand intravascular volume, reduce resuscitation requirements, and limit edema in unburned tissue following a major burn. Fresh frozen plasma appears to be a useful and effective immediate burn resuscitation fluid but its benefits must be weighed against its costs, and risks of viral transmission and acute lung injury. Albumin, in contrast, is less expensive and safer and has demonstrated ability to reduce resuscitation requirements and possibly limit edema-related morbidity.

This article discusses commonly used methods of monitoring and determining the end points of resuscitation. Each end point of resuscitation is examined as it relates to use in critically ill burn patients. Published medical literature, clinical trials, consensus trials, and expert opinion regarding end points of resuscitation were gathered and reviewed. Specific goals were a detailed examination of each method in the critical care population and how this methodology can be used in the burn patient. Although burn resuscitation is monitored and administered using the methodology as seen in medical/surgical intensive care settings, special consideration for excessive edema formation, metabolic derangements, and frequent operative interventions must be considered.

The inflammatory state after burn injury is characterized by an increase in capillary permeability that results in protein and fluid leakage into the interstitial space, increasing resuscitative requirements. Although the mechanisms underlying increased capillary permeability are complex, damage from reactive oxygen species plays a major role and has been successfully attenuated with antioxidant therapy in several disease processes. However, the utility of antioxidants in burn treatment remains unclear. Vitamin C is a promising antioxidant candidate that has been examined in burn resuscitation studies and shows efficacy in reducing the fluid requirements in the acute phase after burn injury.

Children have unique physiologic, physical, psychological, and social needs compared with adults. Although adhering to the basic tenets of burn resuscitation, resuscitation of the burned child should be modified based on the child's age, physiology, and response to injury. This article outlines the unique characteristics of burned children and describes the fundamental principles of pediatric burn resuscitation in terms of airway, circulatory, neurologic, and cutaneous injury management.

Intravenous (IV) cannulation and sterile IV salt solutions may not be options in resource-limited settings (RLSs). This article presents recipes for fluid resuscitation in the aftermath of burns occurring in RLSs. Burns of 20% total body surface area (TBSA) can be resuscitated, and burns up to 40% TBSA can most likely be resuscitated, using oral resuscitation solutions (ORSs) with salt supplementation. Without IV therapy, fluid resuscitation for larger burns may only be possible with ORSs. Published global experience is limited, and the magnitude of burn injuries that successfully respond to World Health Organization ORSs is not well-described.

Failed burn resuscitation can occur at various points. Early failed resuscitation will be largely caused by prehospital factors. During resuscitation, failure will present as a patient's nonresponse to adjunctive therapy. Late failure will occur in the setting of multiple organ dysfunction syndrome.

Burn care providers must be vigilant during the resuscitation to identify a threatened resuscitation so that adjunctive therapies or rescue maneuvers can be used to convert to a successful resuscitation. However, when a patient's resuscitative course becomes unsalvageable, transition to comfort care should be taken to avoid prolongation of suffering.

phase of injury include pharmacologic agents, early enteral nutrition, and the aggressive approach of early excision of large injuries. Recent investigations into the genomic response to severe burns and the application of computer-based decision support tools will likely guide future resuscitation, with the goal of further reducing mortality and morbidity, and improving functional and quality of life outcomes.

CRITICAL CARE CLINICS

Foreword

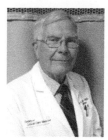

Richard W. Carlson, MD, PhD, MCCM, MACP
Consulting Editor

This issue of *Critical Care Clinics* features a series of informative articles that describe recent advances plus the current status of Burn Resuscitation. I am especially pleased that my colleagues from Maricopa Medical Center and the Arizona Burn Center: Drs Foster, and Caruso, are guest editors for this issue. Critical care clinicians of all stripes will find the information contained in this collection of articles to be of great interest.

This issue will also be the last issue of *Critical Care Clinics* for which I will serve as Consulting Editor. Thirty years ago, I was asked to coedit an issue of *Critical Care Clinics* on Renal Failure and Associated Metabolic Disturbances (Vol. 3(4), October 1987). This led W.B. Saunders to invite me to become Consulting Editor, a position I have enjoyed for nearly three decades. It has been an honor to work with W.B. Saunders, and subsequently, Elsevier, for these many years, and to introduce our readers to multiple editors, authors, and topics. In particular, I would like to thank Mr Patrick Manley and his staff for their guidance and support. It is fitting that Dr John Kellum, an authority on renal and metabolic crises as well as the broad field of Critical Care, will assume the helm as Consulting Editor. Dr Kellum is a distinguished practitioner and researcher whose knowledge and vision will guide the selection of subsequent editors and topics. I wish him and *Critical Care Clinics* continued success. Thank you for the opportunity to serve these many years.

Richard W. Carlson, MD, PhD, MCCM, MACP
Department of Medicine
Maricopa Medical Center
2601 Roosevelt Street
Phoenix, AZ 85008, USA

Mayo Clinic College of Medicine
Scottsdale, AZ, USA

University of Arizona College of Medicine
Phoenix, AZ, USA

E-mail address:
richardw_carlson@dmgaz.org

Crit Care Clin 32 (2016) xiii
http://dx.doi.org/10.1016/j.ccc.2016.08.001
0749-0704/16/© 2016 Published by Elsevier Inc.

Preface

Fluid Resuscitation in Burn Patients: Current Care and New Frontiers

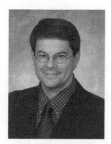 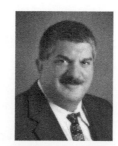

Kevin N. Foster MD, MBA, FACS   Daniel M. Caruso, MD, FACS
Editors

The recognition that burn injury causes a profound inflammatory response accompanied by movement of intravascular fluid into the extravascular space and that this intravascular fluid loss must be aggressively replaced by intravenous fluid administration was one of the key advances in burn care in the last century. Subsequent studies of fluid resuscitation following burn injury demonstrated improved patient outcomes. Since that time, fluid resuscitation in burn patients has been a fertile field for both basic science and clinical research.

Current clinical care for fluid resuscitation of burned patients consists of determining the extent of the burn injury, determining the volume or rate of fluid administration based on one of several validated fluid formulas, and administering fluid as a balanced salt solution with or without colloid. There is no recognized specific standard of care for burn resuscitation. Subsequent fluid administration is based on patient response, primarily urine output. Additional modifications to the fluid resuscitation strategy may be made based on individual patient characteristics such as delayed presentation and resuscitation, the presence of inhalation injury, the presence of comorbidities such as cardiac and/or pulmonary disease, and the development of conditions such as acute kidney injury.

This issue of *Critical Care Clinics* reviews the current status of fluid resuscitation in burn patients, including existing knowledge of the pathophysiologic mechanisms of burn shock, the use of colloid in resuscitation paradigms, monitoring the success of fluid resuscitation, and fluid resuscitation in pediatric patients. Additional topics to be covered include the utility of vitamin C in acute resuscitation, caring for patients with complicated resuscitations, treatment options when standard clinical fluid resuscitation paradigms fail, and the recent issue of so-called fluid creep and overaggressive resuscitation. Finally, this issue also presents the relatively novel concept of

Crit Care Clin 32 (2016) xv–xvi
http://dx.doi.org/10.1016/j.ccc.2016.07.001
0749-0704/16/© 2016 Published by Elsevier Inc.

protocolized and/or computerized models of resuscitation and explores novel and unique future therapies in burn resuscitation.

Kevin N. Foster, MD, MBA, FACS
The Arizona Burn Center
University of Arizona College of Medicine
2601 East Roosevelt
Phoenix, AZ 85008, USA

Daniel M. Caruso, MD, FACS
Department of Surgery
University of Arizona College of Medicine
The Arizona Burn Center
Maricopa Medical Center
2601 East Roosevelt
Phoenix, AZ 85008, USA

E-mail addresses:
kevin_foster@dmgaz.org (K.N. Foster)
danile_caruso@dmgaz.org (D.M. Caruso)

Introduction: Burn Resuscitation

 CrossMark

Kevin N. Foster, MD, MBA

Fluid resuscitation after thermal injury has been recognized as an essential component in burn care for the last half century. Indeed, implementation of fluid resuscitation protocols is one of the first true advances in care of thermally injured patients, resulting in decreased morbidity and increased survival. Although appropriate fluid resuscitation after thermal injury unquestionably leads to better patient outcomes, and several aspects of fluid resuscitation are widely accepted, many methodologic areas of uncertainty and even contention remain to be better defined. There is no one true method of burn resuscitation accepted by all burn care professionals. The objectives of this series of articles are to identify the important components of burn fluid resuscitation including those of controversy, review the existing literature in these areas, identify best practices where they exist, and suggest where future research should be focused. The overall goal is to improve fluid resuscitation of the thermally injured patient and maximize positive patient outcomes.

A key to managing burn injury fluid resuscitation is understanding the pathophysiologic processes involved in burn shock. Thermal injury induces a massive acute inflammatory response that has both adaptive and maladaptive aspects. There is release of mediators that act locally at the injured site and distally beyond the burn injury. There is a change in capillary permeability and massive fluid shifts from one body compartment to another. These changes necessitate the large volume fluid resuscitation characteristic of burn injury. Lack of or inadequate resuscitation leads to organ dysfunction and often death. On the other hand, overaggressive resuscitation leads to edema and other potential problems. Finally, recognizing the causative components of burn shock provides areas of research and possible therapeutic intervention.

The need for fluid resuscitation after burn injury is a well-recognized phenomenon in burn care. What is not known and what is a point of significant current controversy is the best method of fluid resuscitation. Specifically, there is debate over the use of colloids during acute resuscitation. The benefits of colloid administration include expansion of intravascular volume, reduction in the total amount of fluid needed for resuscitation, and decreased edema. Presumably, appropriate use of colloid should also result in better patient outcomes. However, colloid use is not without potential adverse effects. This issue explores the existing literature on colloid use in burn resuscitation and offers areas for further investigation.

An important aspect for any therapeutic intervention is the need for evaluation and re-evaluation of the success or failure of that intervention. This is particularly true for

Disclosure Statement: The author has nothing to disclose.
The Arizona Burn Center, Maricopa Integrated Health Systems, 2601 East Roosevelt, Phoenix, AZ 85008, USA
E-mail address: Kevin_foster@dmgaz.org

Crit Care Clin 32 (2016) 489–490
http://dx.doi.org/10.1016/j.ccc.2016.06.011
0749-0704/16/© 2016 Elsevier Inc. All rights reserved.

fluid resuscitation in burn patients. Traditionally, the adequacy of fluid administration had been monitored by urine output. Indeed, most current fluid resuscitation protocols are based on patient urine output. However, it is possible that additional monitoring methods may augment fluid resuscitation protocols. Additionally, burn patients with existing renal dysfunction or burn patients who experience acute kidney injury as a result of their burn cannot be monitored effectively by urine output alone, and other methods must be used. This issue reviews the various techniques of monitoring resuscitation.

One of the few novel therapeutic interventions trialed in burn resuscitation is the use of vitamin C. Reactive oxygen species likely cause damage after thermal injury. Attenuation of this damage may be mediated by exogenous antioxidants such as vitamin C. This issue reviews the use and utility of vitamin C as an adjunct to burn fluid resuscitation.

Thermal burns are a fairly common injury in children. Resuscitation of these burned children is different than in burned adults. Pediatric burn patients have unique pathophysiology, and fluid resuscitation must be modified to meet these needs. This issue explores different requirements and interventions in fluid resuscitation of pediatric burn patients.

Unfortunately, thermal injury is common in areas of low socioeconomic status and limited resources. Fluid resuscitation of patients in these environments is particularly challenging. This issue describes treatment options for fluid resuscitation in austere environments in which resources taken for granted in developed countries are limited or absent.

Burn resuscitation formulas have existed for decades and have been used successfully in many patients. Unfortunately, some burn resuscitations are complicated by preexisting or new-onset disease processes, which make standard resuscitation impossible. These conditions include heart disease, liver failure, acute or chronic renal dysfunction, inhalation injuries, and others. This issue describes the common complications seen in burn resuscitation and offers treatment options for these complicated patients.

One recently recognized complication associated with burn resuscitation is the concept of fluid creep defined as overzealous administration of crystalloid during acute resuscitation of burn patients. This issue explores this phenomenon and offers techniques to avoid it.

The methodology involved in burn fluid resuscitation has remained largely unchanged since the introduction of resuscitation formulas more than 50 years ago. This article describes potential future therapies to improve burn fluid resuscitation.

Burn resuscitation is found to be highly successful when protocols are implemented and followed appropriately. Burn fluid resuscitation, thus, lends itself nicely to electronic and computerized management strategies. This issue describes the use of protocolized resuscitation modalities in burn fluid resuscitation.

The Physiologic Basis of Burn Shock and the Need for Aggressive Fluid Resuscitation

CrossMark

Lisa Rae, MD[a],*, Philip Fidler, MD[b], Nicole Gibran, MD[c]

KEYWORDS

- Burn • Thermal injury • Shock • Resuscitation • Inflammation • SIRS • Edema
- Hypovolemia

KEY POINTS

- The inflammatory responses to burn injury cause multiorgan failure and early death without adequate resuscitation.
- Inflammatory mediator's effects on endothelial and smooth muscle cells result in leakage of fluid from the intravascular to extravascular space at the site of the burned tissue, and systemically in all organs leading to hypovolemic shock.
- Resuscitation causes edema, which contributes to morbidity and mortality in the thermally injured patient.
- Reactive oxygen species produced by injured tissue contributes to the inflammatory response.
- Nitric oxide production after injury potentiates endothelial leak, contributing to hypotension and poor organ perfusion.

INTRODUCTION

Burn trauma in the current age of medical care still portends a 3% to 8% mortality. Of patients who die from their burn injuries, 58% of deaths occur in the first 72 hours after injury, indicating death from the initial burn shock.[1] Significant thermal injury incites an inflammatory response, which distinguishes burns from other trauma. Since World War I, human and animal studies have brought us closer to understanding the unprecedented inflammatory reaction caused by burn injury. Rapid and extensive fluid shifts in burned and nonburned tissue result in progressive hypovolemia, peripheral edema, multiorgan failure, and death.[2–4] Capillary leak both locally and systemically causes complications from edema and fluid overload.[5] Research efforts have been focused

Disclosure Statement: Nothing to disclose.
[a] Department of Trauma, Surgical Critical Care and Emergency General Surgery, Vanderbilt University Medical Center, 1211 21st Avenue South, MAB 404, Nashville, TN 37212, USA; [b] Swedish Hospital, 601 E. Hampden Avenue, Englewood, CO 80113, USA; [c] UW Burn Center, 325 9th Avenue, Seattle, WA 98104, USA
* Corresponding author.
E-mail address: Lisa.Rae@vanderbilt.edu

Crit Care Clin 32 (2016) 491–505
http://dx.doi.org/10.1016/j.ccc.2016.06.001
0749-0704/16/$ – see front matter © 2016 Elsevier Inc. All rights reserved.

criticalcare.theclinics.com

on resuscitation to ameliorate burn shock, multiorgan failure, and the surge of inflammatory mediators to improve morbidity and mortality. The inflammatory mediators of burned skin trigger a systemic response that alters cardiovascular function, including macrocirculation and microcirculation, and pulmonary, hepatic, renal, gastrointestinal, and endocrine function. This article focuses on the current understanding of the pathophysiology of burn shock, the inflammatory response, and the direction of research and targeted therapies to improve resuscitation, morbidity, and mortality. Despite improvements in critical care and burn survival, a recent study showed that the greatest burden of mortality from burn is still burn shock and failure of initial resuscitation.[1] Of those who died of thermal injury, 55% died within 72 hours, 36% died of burn shock defined as acute functional hypoperfusion, and 28% died of subsequent multiorgan failure or sepsis.

PROGRESSION OF BURN SHOCK AND MULTIORGAN DYSFUNCTION

Shock is defined as inadequate oxygen delivery to meet the metabolic demands of the tissues; this leads to organ dysfunction and eventually failure. Mortalities increase with the number of failing organ systems. The development of multiorgan dysfunction syndrome (MODS) due to sepsis is well established; it is also clear that systemic inflammatory responses can lead to MODS in the absence of infection.[6]

The physiology of burn injury is well recognized as a model of sterile shock and a clear cause for the development of MODS, distinguishing systemic inflammatory response syndrome (SIRS) from sepsis.[7] A study of thermally injured patients was performed evaluating the severity of organ failure with outcomes. An organ failure scale was applied to 529 burn patients; the scale ranged from 0 to 6 (0, no organ dysfunction; 6, organ failure) for each of 6 organ systems. Of the 93.7% of patients who survived, the mean organ failure score was 3.2 compared with 23.1 in nonsurvivors. A mortality of approximately 50% correlated with an organ failure score of greater than 14.[8] In the pediatric burn population, a study was conducted to assess the incidence of multiple organ failure and outcomes. Denver 2 scores were used to assess the degree of organ dysfunction. Increased burn size and depth of burn were correlated with increased incidence of organ failure as well as increased incidence of infection and sepsis. Respiratory failure was most common, followed by cardiac, hepatic, and renal failure. Although the incidence of hepatic or renal failure may be less, this resulted in mortality more frequently.[9] Lactic acidosis and elevated base deficit (BD) levels are well-established markers of inadequate tissue oxygenation and progressive organ dysfunction and portend worse outcomes in the critically ill. In a study of 38 severely burned patients with mean total burn surface area (TBSA) of 36% ± 15%, a BD less than −6 mmol/L in the first 24 hours after burn correlated with increased incidence of acute respiratory distress syndrome (ARDS) and MODS.[10] Another study evaluating BD and lactate levels during burn resuscitation confirmed increased mortality with increased BD and lactate derangement. As well, they noted that normalization of BD within 24 hours after burn injury correlated with improved outcomes compared with those with prolonged elevated BD.[11] These findings have been corroborated in other studies in burn patients.[12,13] Therefore, it can be concluded that increased tissue hypoxia may represent underresuscitation and result in increased organ dysfunction and higher mortalities.

BURN EDEMA AND HYPOVOLEMIA

Burn shock results from the loss of intravascular fluid, because proteins and plasma are sequestered in burned and nonburned tissues. Observed fluid shifts triggered by local and systemic mediators of inflammation result in endothelial leak and profound hypovolemia. However, fluid replacement alone does not ameliorate the effects of burn shock.[7] Resuscitation efforts to prevent hypovolemic shock, tissue hypoxia, and multiorgan failure are complicated by significant edema in all tissues leading to complications of respiratory failure, abdominal compartment syndrome, ocular and extremity compartment syndromes, which result in significant morbidity and mortality.[14–19] Therefore, resuscitation is not as simple as replacing fluid lost from the intravascular space.

An understanding of the microvascular fluid balance and exchange is necessary to understand the changes that occur after burn injury. The Starling equation describes the forces at the level of the capillary that maintain intravascular volume and prevent edema formation in the normal physiologic state (**Fig. 1**).

The Starling equation is as follows:

$$Q = K_f (P_c - P_i) + \sigma (\pi_c - \pi_i)$$

where Q is the net fluid filtration rate across the capillary from the intravascular space to the interstitium; K_f is the fluid filtration coefficient; K_f describes the ability of fluid to exit the capillary into the interstitium and is influenced by the surface area of the capillary bed and the compliance of the interstitial space; P_c is the capillary hydrostatic pressure promoting fluid to flow out of the capillary; P_i is the interstitial hydrostatic

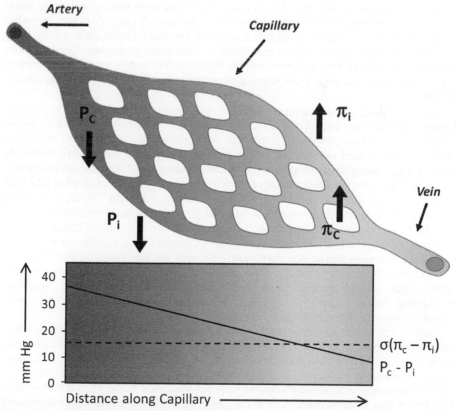

Fig. 1. Starling forces across the capillary bed.

pressure; σ is the coefficient of capillary permeability; π_c is the plasma oncotic pressure; and π_c is the interstitial oncotic pressure. The amount of fluid that crosses from the capillary to the interstitium, Q, is normally taken up by the lymphatics.[20,21]

Hyaluronic acid, collagen, and proteoglycans provide the structural integrity of the interstitial space and exist in a coiled state providing a negative elastic force (**Fig. 2**). When this extracellular matrix is disrupted, the forces limiting the influx of fluid are lost. As the tissues become edematous, the compliance of the tissue increases such that volume increases more rapidly than pressure. The interstitial matrix uncoils, increasing the compliance of the interstitium further, allowing dramatic efflux of fluid into the extravascular space and promoting edema formation.[22,23]

In normal tissue, a 20 to 25 mm Hg gradient between the plasma and interstitial oncotic pressure causes fluid to resorb back into the intravascular space. However, in burned tissue, this gradient approaches zero or may even become negative, drawing fluid out of the vasculature and into the interstitium.[24] Direct measurement in sheep after 70% TBSA burn showed a rapid decrease in interstitial hydrostatic pressure (P_i) from -2 to -11 mm Hg in the first 5 minutes. At the same time, the plasma oncotic pressure declined from 16 to 10 mm Hg over 6 hours. Therefore, the rapid and sustained edema formation after burn results from both increased interstitial compliance and declining plasma oncotic pressure. This study also showed that nonburned skin became edematous once resuscitation was initiated and the plasma oncotic pressure was decreased.[24] Another study demonstrated protein translocation from the intravascular to extravascular space to increase 100-fold in burned tissues and 5-fold in nonburned tissues at the time of burn injury.[25] Studies have shown increased water content in nonburned tissues with as little as a 10% burn.[26] Leape[27] noted an immediate increase in radiolabeled albumin movement into the interstitium in a 50% body surface area burn. Two potential mechanisms have been proposed. One suggests protein washout from the capillaries into the tissues and therefore increased interstitial oncotic pressure. The other cites increased capillary permeability (σ) in the nonburned tissues.

An in vitro study using murine endothelium to investigate the progression of endothelial leak after burn injury used a monolayer of endothelial cells treated with serum from burned rats compared with sham rats. An increased endothelial leak was noted in monolayers treated with burned rat serum. Treatment of the cells with granulocyte macrophage colony stimulating factor (GM-CSF) caused significant decrease in endothelial leakage when challenged with serum from burned rats,[28] suggesting GM-CSF may be part of the compensatory anti-inflammatory response. Studies detecting interleukin-1 (IL-1) and IL-1 receptor antagonist (IL-1ra) showed immediate increased circulating levels after burn in a dose-dependent manner, with higher concentrations in larger TBSA burns and increased area of full-thickness burns. Furthermore, levels of IL-1 and IL-1ra were higher in patients with infectious complications as well.[29] Knowledge of the inflammatory mediators that result in increased endothelial leak, hypovolemic shock, and multiorgan failure in the burn patient has increased. However, modulating these factors to improve resuscitation, dampen the inflammatory response, and decrease multiorgan failure remains elusive.

There is a dose-response curve between the size of the burn and the length of time until tissue edema is at its maximum. Carvajal and colleagues[30] demonstrated that peak burn edema in a 10% burn occurred at 3 hours, whereas in a 40% burn, peak edema formation occurred at 12 hours. Other studies have noted edema formation occurs more rapidly in a partial-thickness than full-thickness burns.[30–32] It is theorized that this is due to destruction of the capillary bed underlying a full-thickness burn, and therefore, endothelial leak–driven edema is lessened. In line with this theory,

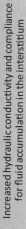

Edema formation is rapid in the first 1–2 h

| Sustained increased capillary permeability in the burn wound | Immediate increase in fluid and protein across the capillary to the interstitial space | Transient increase in capillary hydrostatic pressure in the burn wound |

Loss of integrity in the interstitial space

| Disruption of collagen and hyaluronic acid scaffolding | Progressive increased interstitial space compliance with edema formation | Increased hydraulic conductivity and compliance for fluid accumulation in the interstitium |

Loss of oncotic gradient between the plasma and interstitium

| Loss of plasma proteins results in a vacuum effect of fluid from the intravascular space to the interstitial space | Decreased function of the capillaries and lymphatics especially in full-thickness burns cannot maintain fluid and protein balance |

Progressive intravascular fluid loss and hypovolemia

| Resuscitation required to prevent multiorgan failure and cardiovascular collapse | Edema formation is exaggerated by fluid resuscitation |

Fig. 2. Pathophysiology of burn edema and progressive hypovolemia.

the rate of resorption from lymphatics is also faster in partial-thickness rather than full-thickness burns. The difference in the rates of resorption is thought to be due to the destruction of lymphatics in full thickness compared with partial thickness burns, where the lymphatics are still patent (**Table 1**). Studies on edema formation and resorption demonstrate rapid edema formation over the first 4 hours with peak edema at 12 hours.[20] This is not to suggest that the endothelial leak has closed; edema formation continues, but clearance by lymphatics is upregulated and produces a steady state by 12 to 18 hours after burn. Without resuscitation, multiorgan failure and cardiovascular collapse would result. However, edema formation is exaggerated by resuscitation due to the endothelial leak and vasodilation-driven intravascular volume depletion and hypovolemia.[31] Whereas most resuscitations proceed well, decreasing complications of fluid overload during burn resuscitation continues to be a problem for some patients and remains the focus of ongoing research.

MULTIORGAN DYSFUNCTION AFTER BURN INJURY

Decreased cardiac output represents one of the earliest responses to burn injury despite adequate fluid resuscitation with studies indicating that the mechanisms are unrelated to intravascular fluid loss and hypovolemia.[4] Studies have shown that cardiac output is improved by fluid resuscitation but does not fully restore left ventricular contractility with maximal preload and coronary blood flow.[33,34] Studies in adult guinea pigs with burn size greater than 45% TBSA demonstrated changes in cardiac function, including impaired isovolumetric relaxation and diastolic compliance as well as decreased left ventricular contractility.[34] Elevated troponin I levels have been detected after burn in both animals and humans. Elevated troponin I levels were noted in humans with greater than 20% TBSA burn for 12 hours after thermal injury, adding to the evidence of burn-induced cardiac injury.[35] Of note, elevated troponin I levels were not detected in burns less than 10% TBSA. Further studies regarding the timing of myocardial deficits after burn injury have demonstrated myocardial dysfunction beginning as early as 2 hours after burn with resolution between 48 to 72 hours.[36] Studies by Horton have elucidated many of the mechanisms that result in the

Table 1 Differences in tissue response to partial and full-thickness burn injury		
	Partial Thickness Burn	**Full Thickness Burn**
Tissue perfusion	Initial vasoconstriction causing transient decreased dermal blood flow	Vascular occlusion causing prolonged decrease in blood flow
Capillary permeability	Increased permeability after dermal vessel injury	Increased after injury to patent dermal and subdermal vessels
Edema formation	In dermis and junction between epidermis-dermis	In dermis and subdermis
Interstitial change	Loss of interstitial matrix in burned areas with maintained tissue integrity in nonburned dermis	Loss of interstitial integrity and damage to matrix components, hyaluronic acid, and collagen
Interstitial pressure	Mild decreased in injured dermis	Marked decrease in injured dermis
Lymphatics	Preserved function allowing for rapid clearance of edema and lost proteins	Damaged with severely impaired clearance of edema and lost proteins

observed cardiac dysfunction after burn injury. Tumor necrosis factor-α (TNF-α), IL-1β, and IL-6 have all been found in elevated concentrations in serum of thermally injured patients compared to normal controls.[39] Administration of TNF-α to healthy volunteers induces changes in cardiac function similar to those seen in burn patients or other trauma.[37] To further evaluate the role of TNF-α in after-burn cardiac dysfunction, Giroir and colleagues[38] showed increased TNF-α and decreased myocardial contractility in guinea pigs with 40% TBSA burns, and demonstrated improvement with anti-TNF-α. Horton and colleagues[39] evaluated the role of antioxidants on cardiomyocytes in multiple small animal models and their effects on inflammatory cytokines TNF-α, IL-1β, and IL-6. Vitamins A, C, E, and Zinc resulted in recovery of myocardial contractility compared with the control group who developed impaired left ventricular contraction and increased preload. It was further demonstrated that the antioxidant-treated group had decreased nuclear translocation of nuclear factor-κB (a DNA transcription factor) leading to decreased production of inflammatory cytokines by the cardiomyocyte.[39] Evaluation of IL-1β and TNF-α in human studies has not shown the same correlations; fluctuating levels were seen throughout the hospital course and were poor predictors for clinical changes or outcomes.[29,40]

Another potential player in the resulting myocardial dysfunction seen in burn trauma may be apoptosis or programmed cell death. A comparison of myocardial function and the number of apoptotic cells in the heart after 40% TBSA full-thickness burn in rats demonstrated increased left ventricular apoptosis at 24 hours after burn with persistent elevation at 48 hours. Of note, the subendocardial tissue of the left ventricle was the predominant site of apoptotic cells with correlation between the extent of apoptosis and left ventricular pressure dysfunction in the treatment group.[41] Several signal transduction pathways and mechanisms for inflammatory mediators have been described to help explain the myocardial dysfunction associated with burn injury. Which factors are more or less important or may serve as a target for therapy has yet to be determined as well as the roles of locally produced inflammatory mediators that act in an autocrine or paracrine fashion compared with the systemic circulating cytokines.[41–43]

The early effects of burn trauma on organ function and their mechanisms are reviewed to further the understanding of the systemic response to burn injury and the magnitude of the resulting burn shock. Jeschke and colleagues[44] performed an analysis of 242 severely burned children (TBSA >30%), evaluating long- and short-term changes in endocrine, cardiac, musculoskeletal, and hepatic function. Inflammatory markers were evaluated with serum proteome analysis as well.[44] Blood and urine were collected at admission, preoperatively, and 5 days postoperatively to analyze inflammatory cytokine and hormone profiles. Liver size was measured with ultrasound and compared with predicted size for each patient. Resting energy expenditure was measured with indirect calorimetry, and an average increase to 130% of normal was seen immediately after burn injury. Statistically significant increases on after-burn day 1 were noted in complement C3, α2-microglobulin, haptoglobin, and C-reactive protein. Constitutively, active hepatic proteins were significantly decreased on after-burn day 1, including prealbumin, transferrin, apolipoprotein A1. Evaluation of hormone changes due to burn demonstrated both serum glucose and insulin were increased starting on after-burn day 1. Insulin-like growth factor-1 was drastically decreased on day 1 after injury, along with thyroxine and parathyroid hormone, whereas serum and urine cortisol increased significantly. This study demonstrates the complexity and ubiquity of the systemic response to burn injury. The cytokine profile demonstrated dramatic increases in IL-2, IL-4, IL-10, GM-CSF, interferon-γ, IL-5, IL-13, IL-17, IL-6, IL-8, TNF-α, IL-1β, monocyte chemotactic protein 1 (MCP-1), and macrophage inflammatory protein. The significance and role of each of these cyto-kines have yet to be fully understood. Liver size at 1 and 2 weeks after burn increased to 180% and 220%, respectively, of predicted size.[44,45] These findings have added to the overall understanding of the complexity of the physiologic response to burn injury and demonstrated the prolonged time course that persists after burn trauma. Improved understanding of the complexity of the systemic response to burn injury al-ludes to the challenges of intervening in this cascading interdependent system. Ther-apies targeting any one of these factors may result in multiple helpful and/or harmful downstream events.

Because of the evidence that cardiac output decreases after burn injury, studies into the changes in hepatic and intestinal blood flow were undertaken.[46] Uptake of 201 Thallium and Iodine-125-labeled fatty acid was used to assess blood flow to the liver, stomach, small intestine, and kidneys in animals with 20% TBSA scald burns. The Thallium uptake in the kidney was diminished at the 15-minute time point ($P<.01$). However, there was no difference in uptake in the liver or small bowel. Therefore, the hepatic changes noted after burn injury are not the result of ischemia despite changes in cardiac output and renal blood flow. The incidence of acute renal failure (ARF) in burn patients ranges from 4.7% to 28% in recent studies, with varying defini-tions,[47–50] and is associated with increased mortalities from 25% to 75%. Mortality in thermally injured patients who develop ARF improved from 100% to 56% in a study in 1998 as a result of improvements in fluid resuscitation.[49] Since then, factors associ-ated with the development of ARF have been more difficult to identify. In a study by Mosier and colleagues,[48] the development of early ARF was not associated with dif-ferences in volume of resuscitation per weight and TBSA burned or urine output during resuscitation. However, early development of ARF was associated with increased BD in the first 24 hours after burn injury. Furthermore, there are data to suggest that the degree of BD and serum lactate levels are a marker for the degree of inflammatory response.[10,51] This suggests that further improvements in renal function, morbidity, and mortality are dependent on modulating the systemic inflammatory response to burn injury potentially over local or independent organ function.

INFLAMMATORY CYTOKINES AND MEDIATORS OF BURN INJURY

The SIRS exists on a continuum that can mimic physiologic changes in vital signs after running up the stairs, with increased heart rate and respiratory rate, and extend to hy-potension, multiorgan failure, and death. Although burn patients are at high risk for infection, the fever, tachycardia, and hypotension seen early after thermal injury are most commonly due to the inflammatory response to the burn itself and not sepsis. There is great overlap of inflammatory mediators after burn injury (SIRS) and sepsis, making it difficult to clinically differentiate and treat the 2 entities appropriately. Sepsis is defined as evidence of infection in the setting of life-threatening organ dysfunc-tion.[52,53] Because the systemic response to burn injury does not distinguish burn shock from sepsis, an alternate definition of burn sepsis has been proposed. The defi-nition is primarily based on clinical evaluation, and it states, sepsis is a change in the burn patient that triggers the concern of infection. It is a presumptive diagnosis whereby antibiotics are started and the search for an underlying cause of infection is initiated.[54]

One study attempted to answer this question using the data collected from the In-flammatory and Host Response to Injury program (Glue Grant), which collected longi-tudinal, prospective data from burn and trauma patients.[55] Sweeney and colleagues[55] evaluated differential gene expression in patients with SIRS following trauma and patients with sepsis to determine whether there is a signature profile that can distinguish SIRS from sepsis; a set of 11 genes was noted to be differentially expressed in SIRS versus sepsis with an area under the curve of 0.83. Evaluation of the identified downstream effects of these genes did not correlate with a set of transcription pathways. TNF-α and known interleukins, unregulated in burn shock, were not specific to SIRS versus sepsis.[55] Another study using Glue Grant data analyzed the proteome and cytokine profiles of severely injured burn survivors compared with nonsurvivors.[56] Of the 22 cytokines tested, statistically significantly elevated levels of IL-4, IL-8, GM-CSF, and MCP-1 were found in the nonsurvivor group; furthermore, 43 proteins involved in inflammation, cell signaling and movement, cell death, tissue development, and the hematologic, lymphatic, and immune systems were found to be significantly different in survivors versus nonsurvivors.[56] Downstream pathways of these proteins included the coagulation cascade, hepatic acute-phase response, the complement cascade, and inflammatory pathways. A study of severely burned pediatric patients also demonstrated marked increased IL-8, MCP-1, GM-CSF, and IL-6. These markers were also associated with increased infections and sepsis during their hospital course.[44,57] As stated previously, these markers do not distinguish SIRS from sepsis. Furthermore, using these as targets to quell the inflammatory response may result in an altered response to infection.

Nitric Oxide

Nitric oxide (NO) has been shown in many studies to alter vascular endothelium and change vasomotor tone in response to inflammation; this is seen in after-burn injury as well.[58] NO is produced when L-arginine is oxidized by the enzyme, nitric oxide synthase (NOS). NO has both local and systemic effects as a potent vasodilator. The effects of NO in different tissues has been studied and noted to be tissue specific. In the gastrointestinal tract after thermal injury, studies have shown an increase in mucosal NOS activity leading to increased mucosal permeability and bacterial translocation; this finding was suppressed by an NOS inhibitor.[59] Reduction in pulmonary vascular permeability by NOS inhibition was demonstrated in sheep with a 40% TBSA burn and inhalation injury; however, this was not seen in the vasculature of the burned tissue. Still, sheep treated with the inhibitor of NOS did require less fluid resuscitation than the control.[60] Another study demonstrated that inhaled NO after inhalation injury in sheep resulted in decreased lung water content, decreased pulmonary vascular resistance, increased reflection coefficient, compared with the control inhalation injury group.[61] Circulating and urinary levels of NO byproducts appear to increase in a dose-dependent manner with increased burn size. However, production of NO was significantly depressed in the nonsurvivor group compared with survivors.[62–64] This may indicate that although NO increases endothelial leak and morbidity because of fluid overload and tissue edema, its function may be necessary for survival. In other studies evaluating inducible NO production after burn injury, administration of NOS inhibitor has been shown to decrease edema in the burned tissues[65] and fluid leakage from the capillary bed.[66] Whether NO represents a good target to alter microvascular permeability remains unclear.

Oxidative Stress

Oxygen radicals result from a variety of biochemical reactions. Increased production of reactive oxygen species (ROS) results from trauma, including burn injury.[67] These oxygen radicals are released from neutrophils after inflammation or ischemic injury.[68,69] The production of ROS contributes to increased vascular permeability, tissue edema, systemic inflammation, and multiorgan dysfunction.[70–72] In a study comparing oxidative stress in sepsis and nonseptic burn patients, markers of oxidative stress were collected daily for 5 days either after burn injury or after identification of sepsis. There were significant differences from day 1 to 5 in C-reactive protein, which increased in the nonseptic burn patient and decreased in the septic patient. ROS intensity increased over the initial 5 days after burn injury, whereas a relatively constant ROS intensity was found in the septic patients. Initially elevated lactate levels on day 1 decreased over the 5 days of the study in both groups.[73] Using antioxidants to decrease the downstream effects of ROS in burn patients is a potential target for therapy to decrease vascular permeability and eventual organ dysfunction. Several studies in animals have used vitamin C for its antioxidant properties with promising results by demonstrating decreased fluid requirements for resuscitation.[74,75] In clinical trials, the results are not as clear.[76,77]

Histamine

Tissue destruction as the inciting event after burn injury initiates the inflammatory response. Whereas many cells in the epidermis and dermis contribute to the local inflammatory response, mast cell degranulation induces the neighboring endothelial cells to produce IL-6, IL-8, and MCP-1. Histamine, one of the mast cell–derived mediators, potentiates endothelial leak[78,79] by upregulating prostacyclin and NO, which subsequently induce endothelial cell rounding, allowing for leakage of intravascular fluid into the extravascular space.[80] Histamine incubated on coronary endothelial cells induced IL-6 and IL-8 production in a dose-dependent manner. Furthermore, lipopolysaccharide, known to induce a strong inflammatory response during infection, added to histamine-augmented production of IL-6, IL-8, and MCP-1. Similar results were noted when endothelial cells were incubated with histamine plus TNF-α.[81] There are multiple overlapping cascades of inflammatory mediators that are triggered by burn injury. Identifying a target that will reduce the deleterious effects of inflammation without compromising the ability to fight infection and promote wound healing remains complex and elusive.

Coagulation Cascade

The same factors that initiate inflammation after burn injury simultaneously activate the extrinsic coagulation cascade. Derangements of the coagulation factors associated with disseminated intravascular coagulation (DIC) have been demonstrated in several studies in burn-injured patients.[82] The degree of hypercoagulable state generated by burn injury occurs in a dose-dependent manner correlated with increased burn size. DIC is characterized by activation of the coagulation and fibrinolytic pathways, leading to consumption of coagulation factors and loss of coagulation regulatory proteins. Elevated levels of D-dimers and factor VIII associated with hypercoagulable state have been detected with burn size as low as 6% TBSA. Thrombelastography (TEG) results demonstrate increased α angle and mean amplitude, supporting the burn-induced hypercoagulable state and elevated levels of D-dimers and factor VIII with increasing burn size.[83–85]

Microvascular emboli have been demonstrated in the major organs in approximately 30% of patients with severe burn injury.[86] There is good evidence that activation of coagulation and fibrinolytic pathways and the formation of microemboli contribute to MODS and mortality in the critically ill.[87,88] In a study of 43 thermally injured patients, serum was collected on after-burn day 1 and 7 and analyzed for differences in components of the coagulation and fibrinolytic pathways.[87] Further analysis was performed to evaluate the differences in survivors compared with nonsurvivors in this study. Thermally injured patients exhibit alterations of the coagulation cascade consistent with a transient DIC. The magnitude of these derangements was increased in the nonsurvivors. Fibrin formation and microemboli in the capillary beds of organs could account for the MODS seen in these burn-injured patients.[89] In the setting of a burn injury with activation of SIRS, progressive hypovolemia, and a hypercoagulable state, it is not difficult to understand the impending multiorgan failure and systemic collapse burn patients experience. A study in trauma patients evaluated the incidence of MODS in patients with and without DIC. Patients with DIC had worse outcomes, higher incidence of ARDS, and lower platelets and met SIRS criteria for more hospital days.[90] The dysregulation of the coagulation cascade may be the link between activation of inflammation and the resultant multiorgan failure.

PREVENTION OF BURN SHOCK

Resuscitation efforts should focus on ameliorating the hypovolemia associated with burn shock and maintaining organ perfusion. However, interventions must involve a careful balance between too little and too much fluid because both conditions lead to complications and organ failure. It is clear that mediators of the inflammatory response to burn injury may be good targets to modulate burn shock and ultimately reduce fluid requirements. However, the burn community needs further understanding of the cascade of events that result in multiorgan failure and shock if we are to develop therapeutics that can modulate inflammatory responses to injury and ultimately mitigate multiorgan dysfunction. Over the past 50 years, the understanding has advanced significantly. However, there is still a dire need for multicenter clinical trials to develop strategies that result in improved clinical outcomes.

REFERENCES

1. Swanson JW, Otto AM, Gibran NS, et al. Trajectories to death in patients with burn injury. J Trauma Acute Care Surg 2013;74(1):282–8.
2. Underhill FP. Changes in blood concentration with special reference to the treatment of extensive superficial burns. Ann Surg 1927;86(6):840–9.
3. Cope O, Moore FD. The redistribution of body water and the fluid therapy of the burned patient. Ann Surg 1947;126(6):1010–45.
4. Evans EI, Purnell OJ, Robinett PW, et al. Fluid and electrolyte requirements in severe burns. Ann Surg 1952;135(6):804–17.
5. Pham TN, Cancio LC, Gibran NS. American Burn Association practice guidelines burn shock resuscitation. J Burn Care Res 2008;29(1):257–66.
6. Marshall JC. Inflammation, coagulopathy, and the pathogenesis of multiple organ dysfunction syndrome. Crit Care Med 2001;29(7 Suppl):S99–106.
7. Herndon DN. Total burn care. 4th edition. Edinburgh (United Kingdom): Saunders Elsevier; 2012. p. xvii, 784.
8. Saffle JR, Sullivan JJ, Tuohig GM, et al. Multiple organ failure in patients with thermal injury. Crit Care Med 1993;21(11):1673–83.
9. Kraft R, Herndon DN, Finnerty CC, et al. Occurrence of multiorgan dysfunction in pediatric burn patients: incidence and clinical outcome. Ann Surg 2014;259(2):381–7.
10. Cartotto R, Choi J, Gomez M, et al. A prospective study on the implications of a base deficit during fluid resuscitation. J Burn Care Rehabil 2003;24(2):75–84.
11. Andel D, Kamolz LP, Roka J, et al. Base deficit and lactate: early predictors of morbidity and mortality in patients with burns. Burns 2007;33(8):973–8.
12. Jeng JC, Jablonski K, Bridgeman A, et al. Serum lactate, not base deficit, rapidly predicts survival after major burns. Burns 2002;28(2):161–6.

13. Husain FA, Martin MJ, Mullenix PS, et al. Serum lactate and base deficit as predictors of mortality and morbidity. Am J Surg 2003;185(5):485–91.
14. Singh CN, Klein MB, Sullivan SR, et al. Orbital compartment syndrome in burn patients. Ophthal Plast Reconstr Surg 2008;24(2):102–6.
15. Tuggle D, Skinner S, Garza J, et al. The abdominal compartment syndrome in patients with burn injury. Acta Clin Belg 2007;62(Suppl 1):136–40.
16. Strang SG, Van Lieshout EM, Breederveld RS, et al. A systematic review on intra-abdominal pressure in severely burned patients. Burns 2014;40(1):9–16.
17. Peeters Y, Vandervelden S, Wise R, et al. An overview on fluid resuscitation and resuscitation endpoints in burns: past, present and future. Part 1—historical background, resuscitation fluid and adjunctive treatment. Anaesthesiol Intensive Ther 2015;47:6–14.
18. Cordemans C, De Laet I, Van Regenmortel N, et al. Fluid management in critically ill patients: the role of extravascular lung water, abdominal hypertension, capillary leak, and fluid balance. Ann Intensive Care 2012;2(Suppl 1):S1.
19. Saffle JI. The phenomenon of "fluid creep" in acute burn resuscitation. J Burn Care Res 2007;28(3):382–95.
20. Demling RH. The burn edema process: current concepts. J Burn Care Rehabil 2005;26(3):207–27.
21. Starling EH. On the absorption of fluids from the connective tissue spaces. J Physiol 1896;19(4):312–26.
22. Guyton AC, Coleman TG. Regulation on interstitial fluid volume and pressure. Ann N Y Acad Sci 1968;150(3):537–47.
23. Lund T, Onarheim H, Reed RK. Pathogenesis of edema formation in burn injuries. World J Surg 1992;16(1):2–9.
24. Kinsky MP, Guha SC, Button BM, et al. The role of interstitial starling forces in the pathogenesis of burn edema. J Burn Care Rehabil 1998;19(1 Pt 1):1–9.
25. Bert JL, Bowen BD, Reed RK, et al. Microvascular exchange during burn injury: IV. Fluid resuscitation model. Circ Shock 1991;34(3):285–97.
26. Brouhard BH, Carvajal HF, Linares HA. Burn edema and protein leakage in the rat. I. Relationship to time of injury. Microvasc Res 1978;15(2):221–8.
27. Leape LL. Initial changes in burns: tissue changes in burned and unburned skin of rhesus monkeys. J Trauma 1970;10(6):488–92.
28. Zhao J, Chen L, Shu B, et al. Granulocyte/macrophage colony-stimulating factor attenuates endothelial hyperpermeability after thermal injury. Am J Transl Res 2015;7(3):474–88.
29. Vindenes HA, Ulvestad E, Bjerknes R. Concentrations of cytokines in plasma of patients with large burns: their relation to time after injury, burn size, inflammatory variables, infection, and outcome. Eur J Surg 1998;164(9):647–56.
30. Carvajal HF, Linares HA, Brouhard BH. Relationship of burn size to vascular permeability changes in rats. Surg Gynecol Obstet 1979;149(2):193–202.
31. Demling RH, Mazess RB, Witt RM, et al. The study of burn wound edema using dichromatic absorptiometry. J Trauma 1978;18(2):124–8.
32. Sharar SR, Heimbach DM, Green M, et al. Effects of body surface thermal injury on apparent renal and cutaneous blood flow in goats. J Burn Care Rehabil 1988;9(1):26–30.
33. Adams HR, Baxter CR, Parker JL. Contractile function of heart muscle from burned guinea pigs. Circ Shock 1982;9(1):63–73.
34. Adams HR, Baxter CR, Izenberg SD. Decreased contractility and compliance of the left ventricle as complications of thermal trauma. Am Heart J 1984;108(6):1477–87.

35. Murphy JT, Horton JW, Purdue GF, et al. Evaluation of troponin-I as an indicator of cardiac dysfunction after thermal injury. J Trauma 1998;45(4):700–4.
36. Maass DL, Hybki DP, White J, et al. The time course of cardiac NF-kappaB activation and TNF-alpha secretion by cardiac myocytes after burn injury: contribution to burn-related cardiac contractile dysfunction. Shock 2002;17(4):293–9.
37. Tracey KJ, Beutler B, Lowry SF, et al. Shock and tissue injury induced by recombinant human cachectin. Science 1986;234(4775):470–4.
38. Giroir BP, Horton JW, White DJ, et al. Inhibition of tumor necrosis factor prevents myocardial dysfunction during burn shock. Am J Physiol 1994;267(1 Pt 2): H118–24.
39. Horton JW. Free radicals and lipid peroxidation mediated injury in burn trauma: the role of antioxidant therapy. Toxicology 2003;189(1–2):75–88.
40. Cannon JG, Friedberg JS, Gelfand JA, et al. Circulating interleukin-1 beta and tumor necrosis factor-alpha concentrations after burn injury in humans. Crit Care Med 1992;20(10):1414–9.
41. Lightfoot E Jr, Horton JW, Maass DL, et al. Major burn trauma in rats promotes cardiac and gastrointestinal apoptosis. Shock 1999;11(1):29–34.
42. Horton JW. Left ventricular contractile dysfunction as a complication of thermal injury. Shock 2004;22(6):495–507.
43. Carlson DL, Horton JW. Cardiac molecular signaling after burn trauma. J Burn Care Res 2006;27(5):669–75.
44. Jeschke MG, Chinkes DL, Finnerty CC, et al. Pathophysiologic response to severe burn injury. Ann Surg 2008;248(3):387–401.
45. Jeschke MG. The hepatic response to thermal injury: is the liver important for postburn outcomes? Mol Med 2009;15(9–10):337–51.
46. Carter EA, Tompkins RG, Burke JF. Hepatic and intestinal blood flow following thermal injury. J Burn Care Rehabil 1988;9(4):347–50.
47. Holm C, Jorge S, Neves FC, et al. Acute renal failure in severely burned patients. Burns 1999;25(2):171–8.
48. Mosier MJ, Pham TN, Klein MB, et al. Early acute kidney injury predicts progressive renal dysfunction and higher mortality in severely burned adults. J Burn Care Res 2010;31(1):83–92.
49. Jeschke MG, Barrow RE, Wolf SE, et al. Mortality in burned children with acute renal failure. Arch Surg 1998;133(7):752–6.
50. Mustonen KM, Vuola J. Acute renal failure in intensive care burn patients (ARF in burn patients). J Burn Care Res 2008;29(1):227–37.
51. Cochran A, Edelman LS, Saffle JR, et al. The relationship of serum lactate and base deficit in burn patients to mortality. J Burn Care Res 2007;28(2):231–40.
52. Abraham E. New definitions for sepsis and septic shock: continuing evolution but with much still to be done. JAMA 2016;315(8):757–9.
53. Singer M, Deutschman CS, Seymour CW, et al. The third international consensus definitions for sepsis and septic shock (sepsis-3). JAMA 2016;315(8):801–10.
54. Greenhalgh DG, Saffle JR, Holmes JH 4th, et al. American Burn Association consensus conference to define sepsis and infection in burns. J Burn Care Res 2007;28(6):776–90.
55. Sweeney TE, Shidham A, Wong HR, et al. A comprehensive time-course-based multicohort analysis of sepsis and sterile inflammation reveals a robust diagnostic gene set. Sci Transl Med 2015;7(287):287ra71.
56. Finnerty CC, Jeschke MG, Qian WJ, et al. Determination of burn patient outcome by large-scale quantitative discovery proteomics. Crit Care Med 2013;41(6): 1421–34.

57. Finnerty CC, Jeschke MG, Herndon DN, et al. Temporal cytokine profiles in severely burned patients: a comparison of adults and children. Mol Med 2008; 14(9–10):553–60.
58. Rawlingson A. Nitric oxide, inflammation and acute burn injury. Burns 2003;29(7): 631–40.
59. Chen LW, Hsu CM, Cha MC, et al. Changes in gut mucosal nitric oxide synthase (NOS) activity after thermal injury and its relation with barrier failure. Shock 1999; 11(2):104–10.
60. Soejima K, Traber LD, Schmalstieg FC, et al. Role of nitric oxide in vascular permeability after combined burns and smoke inhalation injury. Am J Respir Crit Care Med 2001;163(3 Pt 1):745–52.
61. Enkhbaatar P, Kikuchi Y, Traber LD, et al. Effect of inhaled nitric oxide on pulmonary vascular hyperpermeability in sheep following smoke inhalation. Burns 2005;31(8):1013–9.
62. Do Rosario Caneira da Silva M, Mota Filipe H, Pinto RM, et al. Nitric oxide and human thermal injury short term outcome. Burns 1998;24(3):207–12.
63. Gamelli RL, George M, Sharp-Pucci M, et al. Burn-induced nitric oxide release in humans. J Trauma 1995;39(5):869–77 [discussion: 877–8].
64. Preiser JC, Reper P, Vlasselaer D, et al. Nitric oxide production is increased in patients after burn injury. J Trauma 1996;40(3):368–71.
65. Yonehara N, Yoshimura M. Interaction between nitric oxide and substance P on heat-induced inflammation in rat paw. Neurosci Res 2000;36(1):35–43.
66. Paulsen SM, Wurster SH, Nanney LB. Expression of inducible nitric oxide synthase in human burn wounds. Wound Repair Regen 1998;6(2):142–8.
67. Han S, Cai W, Yang X, et al. ROS-mediated NLRP3 inflammasome activity is essential for burn-induced acute lung injury. Mediators Inflamm 2015;2015: 720457.
68. McCord JM, Fridovich I. The biology and pathology of oxygen radicals. Ann Intern Med 1978;89(1):122–7.
69. Demling RH, LaLonde C. Early postburn lipid peroxidation: effect of ibuprofen and allopurinol. Surgery 1990;107(1):85–93.
70. Ware LB, Fessel JP, May AK, et al. Plasma biomarkers of oxidant stress and development of organ failure in severe sepsis. Shock 2011;36(1):12–7.
71. Abraham E, Singer M. Mechanisms of sepsis-induced organ dysfunction. Crit Care Med 2007;35(10):2408–16.
72. Montuschi P, Barnes P, Roberts LJ 2nd. Insights into oxidative stress: the isoprostanes. Curr Med Chem 2007;14(6):703–17.
73. Muhl D, Woth G, Drenkovics L, et al. Comparison of oxidative stress & leukocyte activation in patients with severe sepsis & burn injury. Indian J Med Res 2011; 134:69–78.
74. Dubick MA, Williams C, Elgjo GI, et al. High-dose vitamin C infusion reduces fluid requirements in the resuscitation of burn-injured sheep. Shock 2005;24(2): 139–44.
75. Tanaka H, Lund T, Wiig H, et al. High dose vitamin C counteracts the negative interstitial fluid hydrostatic pressure and early edema generation in thermally injured rats. Burns 1999;25(7):569–74.
76. Kahn SA, Beers RJ, Lentz CW. Resuscitation after severe burn injury using high-dose ascorbic acid: a retrospective review. J Burn Care Res 2011;32(1):110–7.
77. Buehner M, Pamplin J, Studer L, et al. Oxalate nephropathy after continuous infusion of high-dose vitamin C as an adjunct to burn resuscitation. J Burn Care Res 2016;37(4):e374–9.

78. Carvajal HF, Brouhard BH, Linares HA. Effect of antihistamine-antiserotonin and ganglionic blocking agents upon increased capillary permeability following burn trauma. J Trauma 1975;15(11):969–75.

79. Friedl HP, Till GO, Trentz O, et al. Roles of histamine, complement and xanthine oxidase in thermal injury of skin. Am J Pathol 1989;135(1):203–17.

80. Madigan M, Zuckerbraun B. Therapeutic potential of the nitrite-generated no pathway in vascular dysfunction. Front Immunol 2013;4:174.

81. Li Y, Chi L, Stechschulte DJ, et al. Histamine-induced production of interleukin-6 and interleukin-8 by human coronary artery endothelial cells is enhanced by endotoxin and tumor necrosis factor-alpha. Microvasc Res 2001;61(3):253–62.

82. Lippi G, Ippolito L, Cervellin G. Disseminated intravascular coagulation in burn injury. Semin Thromb Hemost 2010;36(4):429–36.

83. Park MS, Salinas J, Wade CE, et al. Combining early coagulation and inflammatory status improves prediction of mortality in burned and nonburned trauma patients. J Trauma 2008;64(2 Suppl):S188–94.

84. King DR, Namias N, Andrews DM. Coagulation abnormalities following thermal injury. Blood Coagul Fibrinolysis 2010;21(7):666–9.

85. Lavrentieva A, Kontakiotis T, Bitzani M, et al. Early coagulation disorders after severe burn injury: impact on mortality. Intensive Care Med 2008;34(4):700–6.

86. Wells S, Sissons M, Hasleton PS. Quantitation of pulmonary megakaryocytes and fibrin thrombi in patients dying from burns. Histopathology 1984;8(3):517–27.

87. Gando S, Nanzaki S, Sasaki S, et al. Activation of the extrinsic coagulation pathway in patients with severe sepsis and septic shock. Crit Care Med 1998; 26(12):2005–9.

88. Kollef MH, Eisenberg PR, Shannon W. A rapid assay for the detection of circulating D-dimer is associated with clinical outcomes among critically ill patients. Crit Care Med 1998;26(6):1054–60.

89. Garcia-Avello A, Lorente JA, Cesar-Perez J, et al. Degree of hypercoagulability and hyperfibrinolysis is related to organ failure and prognosis after burn trauma. Thromb Res 1998;89(2):59–64.

90. Gando S, Kameue T, Matsuda N, et al. Combined activation of coagulation and inflammation has an important role in multiple organ dysfunction and poor outcome after severe trauma. Thromb Haemost 2002;88(6):943–9.

Colloids in Acute Burn Resuscitation

Robert Cartotto, MD, FRCS(C)[a],*, David Greenhalgh, MD[b]

KEYWORDS

- Burn • Fluid • Resuscitation • Colloids • Shock

KEY POINTS

- Crystalloid excess leading to harm ("fluid creep") has stimulated interest in colloid provision as a volume-sparing strategy.
- Colloids limit edema formation in unburned soft tissues and contribute to reduced resuscitation volumes and faster restoration of cardiac output experimentally.
- Nonprotein colloids are effective volume expanders, but current safety concerns prevent use or recommendation of these colloids in burn resuscitation.
- Fresh frozen plasma is an effective volume-sparing colloid but its benefits must be weighed against its cost and risks of virus transmission and lung injury.
- Albumin has demonstrated volume-sparing effects when used immediately or later in burn resuscitation, possibly leading to improved outcome. It is not known if albumin increases lung extravascular water.

INTRODUCTION

A curious paradox in the acute resuscitation of the burn patient is that debate still continues in 2015 on the use of colloid solutions in burn resuscitation despite the fact that colloids have been recommended components of virtually every burn resuscitation formula since the 1940s (**Table 1**). Uncertainty surrounding the role for colloids and the composition of resuscitation fluids during acute resuscitation has been a repeated theme at Consensus Conferences,[1] at Burn State of the Science Meetings,[2] and in Burn Practice Guidelines of the American Burn Association.[3] A 2010 international survey conducted by the International Society of Burn Injuries and the ABA found that half of respondents initiate colloids in the first 24 hours, with nearly equal preference for fresh frozen plasma (FFP) or albumin as the chosen colloid.[4]

Disclosure Statement: The authors have nothing to disclose.
[a] Department of Surgery, Ross Tilley Burn Centre, Sunnybrook Health Sciences Centre, University of Toronto, Room D712, 2075 Bayview Avenue, Toronto, Ontario M4N 3M5, Canada;
[b] Department of Surgery, Shriners Hospitals for Children Northern California, University of California, Davis, 2425 Stockton Boulevard, Sacramento, CA 95817, USA
* Corresponding author.
E-mail address: robert.cartotto@sunnybrook.ca

Crit Care Clin 32 (2016) 507–523
http://dx.doi.org/10.1016/j.ccc.2016.06.002
0749-0704/16/$ – see front matter © 2016 Elsevier Inc. All rights reserved.
criticalcare.theclinics.com

Table 1
Use of colloids in burn resuscitation formulas 1940 to present

Formula	First 24 h	24–48 h
Harkins Formula[5]	YES (plasma)	Not described
Body Weight Burn Budget[6,7]	YES (stored bank plasma, "plasmanate" [plasma protein fraction], reconstituted 5% albumin)	YES (stored bank plasma, "plasmanate" [plasma protein fraction], reconstituted 5% albumin)
Evans Formula[8]	YES (plasma, plasma substitute [dextran or gelatin], whole blood)	YES (plasma, plasma substitute [dextran or gelatin], whole blood)
Brooke Formula[11]	YES (plasma,[a] dextran, polyvinyl-pyrrolidone, gelatin)	YES (plasma,[a] dextran, polyvinyl-pyrrolidone, gelatin)
Parkland Formula[14]	NO	YES (plasma)
Modified Brooke Formula[16,17]	NO	YES (plasma or "plasma equivalent")
Muir and Barclay Formula[23]	YES (reconstituted dried plasma or dextran)	Not described
Slater Formula[25]	YES (FFP)	Not described
Haifa Formula[24,77]	YES (plasma, "regular plasma")	YES (plasma, "regular plasma")

[a] Discontinued due to concerns surrounding viral hepatitis transmission.

Arguably, equipoise exists as to whether to initiate colloids during acute fluid resuscitation, and if used, the optimal colloid composition, dose, and timing of initiation remain uncertain. The purpose of this article is to review the historical background, physiologic basis, and clinical use of colloids in acute burn resuscitation. This study will not address use of albumin or other colloids after the phase of acute resuscitation to correct hypoalbuminemia.

HISTORICAL PERSPECTIVE

Over the past 7 decades of formula-based burn resuscitation, the use of colloids is best characterized by regular cycles of waxing and waning enthusiasm. Notably, Dr Henry Harkins recommended 1000 cc of plasma for each 10% of the body surface area burned for patients with burns to greater than 10% of their body, in what was probably the earliest burn size–based fluid resuscitation formula (described by Dr I.S. Ravdin and members of the National Research Council in 1942).[5] Following the Coconut Grove disaster in 1942, Cope and Moore[6] proposed a "body weight burn budget" formula that recommended 75 cc of plasma for each 1% of the body surface burned in the first 24 hours and half that amount during the second 24 hours.[6] Later, Moore[7] stated that the total volume of colloid should equal 7.5% of the body weight in the first 24 hours and 2.5% of the body weight in the second 24 hours. Colloid could be provided as stored bank plasma, plasmanate (plasma protein fraction), 5% reconstituted albumin, or smaller quantities of dextran.[7]

This immediate and liberal provision of colloid was based on the observation of hemoconcentration after a major burn, and the deduction that this must have resulted from a loss of plasma volume. Hence, the primary objective was to restore plasma volume with similar fluids. Indeed, the Evans Formula published nearly a decade after the body weight burn budget recommended 1 mL/kg/% total body surface area (TBSA) burn of plasma, plasma substitute, or even whole blood in the first 24 hours after injury and half of that amount between 24 and 48 hours.[8] This colloid volume was equal to the crystalloid volume (0.9% saline) creating a 1:1 colloid to crystalloid ratio.

A subtle alteration occurred 1 year later at the surgical research unit of the Brooke Army Hospital. Recognition that sodium-containing fluid accumulated within burned tissue[9] and that salt solutions alone effectively resuscitated burned rodents,[10] combined with the observations on increased capillary permeability in the burn tissue,[6] led to the belief that "as long as the injured capillaries permit leakage of colloidal particles into the interstitial spaces of burned tissues, the administration of colloid solutions is probably of only limited value in increasing the circulating volume."[11] Accordingly, the Brooke Formula reduced the colloid-to-crystalloid ratio in the first 24 hours to 1:3 by providing 0.5 mL/kg/%TBSA burn of colloid with 1.5 mL/kg/% TBSA burn of lactated Ringer (LR) solution. Concern about transmission of viral hepatitis from plasma also led to the statement that plasma was "never used" and that dextrans, polyvinyl pyrrolidone, and gelatins were equally effective colloids.[11]

By the 1970s, a profound shift away from early provision of colloids had occurred. Dr Carl Moyer and colleagues[12] had successfully resuscitated both scalded dogs and burned humans with LR and no colloid whatsoever and concluded that burn shock arose from an extravascular sodium deficiency that should be treated only with balanced salt solutions. Meanwhile, Drs Baxter and Shires[13,14] had identified both extracellular and intracellular sequestration of sodium and water in burned primates and dogs and recommended correction of these alterations with balanced salt solutions alone in the first 24 hours. Simultaneously, Dr Pruitt and colleagues[15] reported on 10 adult burn patients with burns ranging from 34% to 87% TBSA where the Brooke Formula had been used but with varying colloid content ranging from 0 (no colloid) to 0.5 (half colloid). The study found that "no apparent augmentation of intravascular retention of fluid was observed with increasing colloid content."

Consequently, 2 formulas, both colloid-free in the first 24 hours, emerged and continue as the dominant approaches to burn resuscitation today. Baxter and Shires' Parkland Formula and Pruitt's Modified Brooke Formula recommend, respectively, 4 mL/kg/%TBSA burn and 2 mL/kg/%TBSA burn of LR and no colloids in the first 24 hours. In the second 24 hours, the Modified Brooke Formula provided 0.3 to 0.5 mL/kg/%TBSA burn of "plasma equivalent," "plasma," or "heat-treated plasma product,"[16,17] whereas the Parkland Formula gave 20% to 60% of the calculated plasma volume as stored plasma.[18] Albumin solutions were not specifically described in these formulas even though Janeway and colleagues[19] had reported administration of human albumin (HA) solutions in severely burned patients in 1944. In fact, albumin was the colloid most often used at the US Army Burn Center in the late 1960s and the 1970s (Pruitt BA, personal communication, 2015).

Over the ensuing 4 decades, many variations of the Modified Brooke and Parkland Formulas evolved. These variations included complete abandonment of colloids in the first 48 hours,[20] addition of FFP to the Parkland Formula at 8 hours after burn,[21] or initiation of FFP at 18 to 24 hours.[22] Others recommended the earlier approach of starting colloids immediately using agents such as reconstituted dried plasma or albumin (Muir and Barclay Formula),[23] or plasma (the Haifa Formula),[24] or FFP (the Slater Formula).[25] In fact, surveys have revealed that probably even greater variations existed not only in colloid timing but also in the use of less common nonprotein colloids such as dextran and starches.[2,26]

However, the 1998 Cochrane Injury Group systematic review of 26 controlled trials (3 involving burn patients), which found that albumin-treated patients were at a 6.3% higher risk of death than patients not receiving albumin,[27] and the accompanying headline in the British Medical Journal that albumin was associated with "excessive mortality"[28] caused burn practitioners to use even less albumin and to resort to FFP or even pure crystalloids alone for burn resuscitation at the turn of the millenium.[26,29]

Further reductions in the use of colloids during in burn resuscitation might have continued were it not for Dr Pruitt's perceptive identification of the problem of "fluid creep,"[30] a phenomenon subsequently confirmed by many others,[31–33] which referred to a tendency to administer burn patients excessive amounts of crystalloid fluid that resulted in significant edema-related morbidity. One of several possible causes of fluid creep is thought to be the restriction or outright avoidance of colloids in acute burn resuscitation.[34] This hypothesis has fueled a reawakening of interest in colloid provision as a volume-sparing strategy to address the serious problem of fluid creep. Recent studies suggest that introduction of colloids when actual or projected crystalloid volumes become excessive contributes to improvement in outcomes.[35–38] Although vastly different from the immediate provision of colloids in the early resuscitation formulas,[7,8,11] this "rescue" use of colloids signals a clear shift in philosophy toward the use of more colloids in burn resuscitation.

History—key points

- Resuscitation formulas originally provided colloids immediately to replace observed plasma volume losses.

- Colloid use declined following observations that effective resuscitation could be achieved using crystalloids alone.

- Crystalloid excess leading to harm ("fluid creep") has stimulated interest in colloid provision as a volume-sparing strategy.

RELEVANT PHYSIOLOGY RELATED TO COLLOID RESUSCITATION

It is necessary to examine the various changes in capillary permeability that occur in burned tissue, unburned soft tissue, and the lung in order to understand the basis for, and potential limitation of, colloid use during acute burn resuscitation.

Normal Physiology and Starling Forces

Normally, the distribution of total body water is governed by the interactions between semipermeable vascular membranes, ion pumps, and osmotically active molecules. The Starling model is the basis for the classical model of the capillary membrane described in 1896 by the British physiologist Ernst Starling.[39] This model indicates that a high intravascular pressure is maintained in the circulation without substantial transudation of fluid into the interstitial space (which would collapse the vascular space) because of an opposing osmotic pressure gradient driven by a high intravascular colloid osmotic pressure relative to a lower interstitial colloid osmotic pressure.

The high intravascular colloid osmotic pressure is maintained by macromolecular plasma proteins (most importantly albumin), which are too large to move across the intact capillary membrane to the interstitium in substantial amounts. Thus, the filtration or flux rate (Q) of fluid across the capillary membrane is summarized as:

$$Q = K_f (P_{cap} - P_i) - \sigma (\pi_p - \pi_i)$$

where K_f is the filtration coefficient (a measure of the ease of fluid movement across the membrane), P_{cap} is the capillary hydrostatic pressure, P_i is the interstitial hydrostatic pressure, σ is the reflection coefficient (a measure of the capillary permeability), π_p is the plasma colloid osmotic pressure, and π_i is the interstitial colloid osmotic pressure.

In theory, an adequate intravascular protein concentration with an intact capillary membrane creates an inward force ($\sigma[\pi_p - \pi_i]$) that counterbalances the outward hydrostatic force ($K_f[P_{cap} - P_i]$). In reality, there is always a small amount of fluid flux (Q) and protein movement from the intravascular space into the interstitium. This fluid and protein are continually collected by the lymphatics and eventually returned to the circulation, preventing net fluid and colloid accumulation in the interstitium.[40] This critical role of lymphatics is highly relevant because many of the classical burn experiments on fluid movement and edema are based on the amount of flow and protein content in the lymphatics draining burned tissue, unburned soft tissue, and the lung: Increasing lymphatic flow indicates rising net movement of fluid (Q) from intravascular to interstitium and a rising protein content in the lymph relative to plasma signifies an increase of permeability of the capillary membrane.[41]

As can be deducted from Starling's equation, the variable σ (reflection coefficient) can have a dramatic effect on fluid movement. A value of 1.0 would mean the membrane was impermeable to any macromolecule and would allow the full power of the osmotic gradient ($\pi_p - \pi_i$) to be exerted, whereas a value of 0 would mean the membrane was freely permeable to all molecules, eliminating the osmotic gradient (ie, $0 \times [\pi_p - \pi] = 0$) leaving the hydrostatic gradient unopposed. Thus, when σ drops from its normal value of 0.9 to a lower value (as occurs following mechanical, thermal, or inflammatory injury to the capillary), movement of fluid from intravascular to the interstitium is facilitated.[42]

The entire Starling model may be an oversimplification based on studies on the endothelial glycocalyx (EG), which is the fuzzy layer of glycoproteins that covers the luminal endothelial cell surface. Movement of fluid across the capillary may not be entirely governed by the global difference between intravascular colloid oncotic pressure (π_p) and interstitial colloid osmotic pressure (π_i), but rather by a gradient in osmotic pressure between the surface of the EG and the osmotic pressure just beneath the EG (but still within the vessel proper).[40] This has led to a revised Starling equation:

$$Q = K_f (P_{cap} - P_i) - \sigma (\pi_p - \pi_{GC})$$

where π_{GC} is the colloid osmotic pressure in the subglycocalyx layer.[43] Because π_{GC} is lower than the π_i (used in the original Starling equation), one implication is that filtration (as measured by lymph flow) is less than predicted by the Starling equation, explaining what has been observed experimentally (the "low lymph flow paradox").[43] Another implication arises in situations where the plasma colloid osmotic pressure (π_p) falls (as after burn injury), potentially rendering the osmotic pressure gradient lower than predicted by the classic Starling equation.

Disrupted Physiology After Burns

As early as the 1940s, Cope and Moore[44] and others[45] had demonstrated that there is a profound increase in capillary permeability in acutely burned skin that results from large inflammation-induced gaps between endothelial cells that allow movement of albumin and even much larger plasma proteins along with fluid to leave the intravascular space.[46,47] The increased permeability develops immediately, peaks around 8 hours after burn, and persists more than 48 hours.[41,48–51] It has been estimated that the albumin reflection coefficient in burn tissue drops to 0.3.[52] Consequently, proteins and fluid shift into the interstitial space to create local burn wound edema, and as the burn size approaches 25% TBSA or larger, there is a progressive collapse of the intravascular space, hypoproteinemia, and depression of the plasma colloid osmotic pressure.[41] The capillary leak in the burn tissue is so profound that even immediate resuscitation using colloids such as plasma, dextran, or 6% hetastarch could not establish an effective osmotic gradient and were unable to limit burn tissue edema formation.[50,53,54]

After burns to greater than 25% TBSA, there is also a systemic increase in capillary permeability in unburned soft tissues. However, in contrast to the burn wound, the capillary leak is not as severe, allowing only albumin and smaller plasma proteins to pass,[51] and it is transient, lasting between 6 to 12 hours after burn, after which capillary permeability appears to return to normal.[49,51,55] Although fluid movement from intravascular to interstitial with edema formation starts because of this increase in permeability, after 6 to 12 hours, this process appears to be propagated by the hypoproteinemic state and reduction in the plasma colloid osmotic pressure.[50,51,53] Unlike in the burn wound, resuscitation with colloids, such as plasma or dextran, is able to limit fluid flux into the unburned soft tissue interstitium and helps to restore and maintain a plasma colloid osmotic pressure gradient.[50,53,56]

In the lung unaffected by an inhalation injury, normal capillary permeability appears to be maintained following cutaneous full-thickness burns.[49–51] Fluid flux into the lung interstitium increases immediately after the burn, but this appears to be on the basis of reduced colloid osmotic pressure from the burn-related hypoproteinemic state.[53] Resuscitation using plasma or dextran limited fluid flux into the lung interstitium by generating a colloid osmotic pressure gradient.[50,53]

Finally, compared with using crystalloid, resuscitation with colloids, including dextran, 6% hetastarch, albumin, or plasma, reduced 24-hour resuscitation volumes[53,54] and was associated with more rapid restoration of cardiac output in animal studies.[57,58]

Physiology—key points

- Massive increases in capillary permeability occur in the burn wound, and colloids have no ability to limit fluid flux and edema formation there.

- A systemic but less severe and transient increase in capillary permeability develops in unburned soft tissues after a major burn, but fluid flux and edema accumulation here are due to hypoproteinemia and reduced intravascular colloid osmotic pressure.

- Colloids limit edema formation in unburned soft tissues and contribute to reduced resuscitation volumes and faster restoration of cardiac output experimentally.

CLINICAL RESUSCITATION WITH COLLOIDS

The principle underlying colloid use is that solutions containing macromolecules will theoretically increase plasma colloid osmotic pressure and act as better intravascular volume expanders than crystalloid fluid alone. This section addresses the issues of colloid composition, timing of initiation after burn, and dosage.

Colloid Composition

Nonprotein semisynthetic colloids
Hydroxyethyl starch solutions Hydroxyethyl starch solutions (HES) are colloids that contain large branched chain carbohydrate molecules derived from starches such as corn or potatoes. They are classified by their molecular weight and degree of substitution of glucose molecules for hydroxyethyl (the substitution ratio). The slower

degradation and excretion of HES affords them a longer plasma expansion effect than protein colloids.[59] Current HES formulations, which are eliminated more rapidly, use a lower molecular weight of 130 kDa and have substitution ratios of 0.4 to 0.42, which are respectively abbreviated as HES 130/0.4 (Voluven) and 130/0.42 (Tetraspan).[59]

In burn resuscitation, older studies from the 1980s evaluated moderate- to high-molecular-weight HES such as hetastarch 670/0.75 (Waters and colleagues,[60] N = 26) and pentastarch 250/0.45 (Waxman and colleagues,[61] N = 12). These colloids were initiated around 24 hours after burn after a period of crystalloid resuscitation with LR and were found to be equal to or better than FFP or albumin in terms of their volume expanding and hemodynamic affects. More recently, HES 200/0.6 (Elohaes 6% HES) was evaluated in a randomized trial (n = 26) comparing LR to 2/3 LR and 1/3 HES.[62] The colloid-treated subjects received significantly less fluid and had significantly less body weight gain in the first 24 hours, indicative of the volume and edema-sparing effect of the colloid. Subsequently, a randomized prospective trial compared resuscitation in severely burned adults with LR against a 2:1 combination of LR:HES 130/0.4 but found only a statistically insignificant trend toward less total resuscitation fluid at 24 and 72 hours in the HES + LR group.[63]

Recently, however, large randomized controlled trials (RCTs) among critically ill patients (CHEST and 6S trials)[64,65] identified a significantly increased risk of renal dysfunction requiring renal replacement therapy, significantly more pruritus,[64] and higher 90-day mortality[65] when using HES 130/04[64] or HES 130/0.42[65] compared with crystalloids for fluid resuscitation. Smaller RCTs such as the CRYSTMAS trial also showed a trend toward more frequent need for renal replacement therapy in subjects with severe sepsis that received HES 130/0.4.[66] None of these studies demonstrated any meaningful benefit to HES solutions and consequently some regulatory bodies in Europe have withdrawn HES products,[67] whereas, in the United States, the US Food and Drug Administration has recommended that HES not be used in critically ill patients or those with renal dysfunction.[68] Consequently, HES solutions cannot be recommended for the resuscitation of burn patients at this time.

Gelatins Gelatins were one of the earliest semisynthetic colloids and are obtained from the breakdown of collagen. There are no published clinical trials involving gelatins in burn resuscitation. Historically, gelatins were linked to renal dysfunction and coagulopathy and increased transfusion requirements. A recent systematic review of gelatin for fluid resuscitation found that no statistically significant association could be identified between gelatins and increased mortality or transfusion requirements but the overall effectiveness and safety of gelatins could not be determined.[69]

Dextrans Dextrans are polysaccharides that are available in 3 molecular weights: 10,000, 40,000 (Dextran 40), and 70,000 (Dextran 70). Animal studies have demonstrated that dextrans are effective volume expanders that limit resuscitation requirements and fluid shifts into the unburned soft tissues and lung, minimizing edema formation, compared with crystalloids.[50] When combined with hypertonic saline (7.5% saline Dextran 70), the infusion of hypertonic saline dextran rapidly restored cardiac index, improved urine output, and reduced resuscitation requirements compared with crystalloid alone in the first 8 hours after a 40% full-thickness burn in sheep.[70] However, concerns about dextran-associated anaphylactic reactions, coagulopathy, and possible renal toxicity have limited use of this volume expander in clinical burn resuscitation.

Protein colloids

Fresh frozen plasma FFP is a blood product that has been available since the early 1940s. FFP is collected ("fresh") from a single unit of blood or by apheresis and is then immediately cryopreserved ("frozen") at −30°C and stored for up to 1 year. Originally used as a plasma volume expander, its main use today is in correction of coagulopathy-associated massive bleeding. FFP contains all the plasma proteins (including importantly albumin), all the clotting factors, fibrinogen, electrolytes, and physiologic anticoagulants (protein C, protein S, antithrombin, tissue factor pathway inhibitor).[71] FFP may rarely transmit blood-borne infectious diseases such as HIV (1:7.8 million units), hepatitis C (1:2.3 million units), and hepatitis B (1:153,000 units). The risk of transmission of Creutzfeldt-Jakob disease is uncertain. Also troublesome is FFP's association with transfusion-related acute lung injury (TRALI; 1:10,000 units), which is the commonest cause of a transfusion-related death[71] and which has been reported in burn patients.[72]

FFP use in acute burn resuscitation is typified by Slater Formula developed at the Western Pennsylvania Hospital, in which 2000 mL LR is given over the first 24 hours after burn (83 mL/h) along with 75 mL/kg/36 hours of FFP, but the FFP is titrated to achieve a urinary output of 0.5 to 0.1 mL/kg/h.[25] In a study of patients with burns 30% or more TBSA, immediate resuscitation with LR (4 cc/kg/%TBSA burn), or hypertonic saline (154 meq/L NaCl) or FFP (75 mL/Kg/36 hours) was evaluated. FFP resuscitation required significantly less fluid in the first 24 hours, maintained urine output in the desired range, and was associated with significantly less weight gain after 24 and 48 hours compared with the other 2 regimens.[25] Subsequently, a well-conducted RCT compared resuscitation using the Parkland Formula (n = 15, mean % TBSA burn 50.1) with the Slater Formula (n = 16, mean % TBSA burn 52.1).[73] Resuscitation with FFP achieved the target urinary output goal with significantly less fluid than the crystalloid resuscitation (0.14 L/kg/24 hours vs 0.26 L/kg/24 hours, respectively, $P = .005$). This reduction in fluid volume translated to important improvements in outcome, including significant reductions in weight gain, peak intra-abdominal pressures, and peak inspiratory pressure in the FFP group. Furthermore, adequacy of resuscitation (as measured by the clearance of the base deficit)[74] was significantly greater in the FFP group. This study is of particular importance because it demonstrated that FFP resulted in less fluid administration and that this directly led to clinical benefits.

The Slater Formula was probably derived from the Haifa Formula developed in Israel in the late 1980s.[75,76] This formula was the original description of using 75 mL/kg/36 hours colloid but it used "plasma" not FFP and was subsequently modified to provide 1.5 mL/kg/%TBSA burn/24 hours as "plasma" or "regular plasma" and not FFP, combined with 1.0 mL/kg/%TBSA burn/24 hours of LR.[24,77] In the second 24 hours, half of the first day's colloid is given. The available published reports are retrospective descriptions of the formula, and no study comparing it with a crystalloid control group has been published.

In summary, FFP would appear to be an effective and efficient volume expander for burn resuscitation when used immediately. However, its benefits must be weighed against the cost (about double that for albumin) and risk of disease transmission and TRALI associated with this blood component.

Albumin Albumin is a 67-kDa protein synthesized by the liver with 60% being distributed in the extravascular space and 40% existing in the plasma. The total amount of albumin in a person is approximately 3.5 to 5.0 g/kg or around 250 to 300 g for a 70-kg person.[78] In the healthy person, there is a relatively high amount of leakage of albumin from the intravascular space to the interstitium: approximately 120 to 145 g per day. Almost this entire amount of albumin is returned to the systemic circulation through the lymphatics. The lymphatic system can also increase its flow by a factor of 7 to handle more rapid capillary leak. Typically, albumin will not cross a continuous capillary but will freely flow through sinusoids (liver, bone marrow) or fenestrated capillaries (small intestine, pancreas, adrenal glands). Despite most capillaries having a continuous endothelium, half of the albumin flux occurs through these continuous beds. Active transport, through binding at the surface receptor "abondin," leads to rapid transport across endothelial cell vesicles.[78] Albumin's lifespan is 28 to 36 days, and it is metabolized in skeletal muscle, the liver, and kidney. There is an obligatory loss of roughly 1 g/d into the intestinal tract and a negligible excretion into the urine (a few milligrams per day). Albumin accounts for approximately 50% of the plasma proteins but generates 80% of the plasma colloid on osmotic pressure and, as such, is tremendously important in controlling the distribution and movement of fluid between the body water compartments.[79] Albumin may also contribute to maintaining the intravascular volume as a result of its negative charge. The negative charge may attract cations to help maintain oncotic pressure (the Gibbs-Donnan Effect).[78] Albumin also has an essential role in ligand, metal, and cation binding as well as free radical scavenging and antioxidant functions.[79]

Parenteral HA for infusion is manufactured by Cohn-Oncley cold ethanol fractionation and heat treatment from the plasma of thousands of blood donors. This purification process inactivates known viral pathogens with the exception of nonencapsulated parvovirus B19 (currently plasma donors are screened for parvovirus B19 by nucleic acid testing to reduce this risk).[80] No cases of viral transmission from HA have been recorded.[81] HA is available as an isotonic, iso-oncotic 5% or a hyperoncotic 20% solution, but the electrolyte content (particularly chloride) and buffer vary considerably between manufacturers. In healthy patients, 90% of infused HA remains intravascular 2 hours after transfusion but significantly less is retained in diseased state such as sepsis.[82]

Although HA has been used as a volume expander since the 1940s, its role in fluid resuscitation became very contentious following a Cochrane Injuries Group review in 1998 that found that the use of HA was associated with a pooled increased absolute risk of death of 6% (95% confidence interval [CI]: 3% to 9%).[27] From the standpoint of burn resuscitation, the meta-analysis was quite problematic because, within the burn subgroup, one study was a report on late supplementation of albumin,[83] one RCT involving albumin versus LR was missing,[84] and one study evaluated hypertonic saline-albumin rather than HA alone.[85]

However, confidence in HA's safety has been restored by recent large, pragmatic RCTs among critically ill patients such as the saline versus albumin fluid evaluation (SAFE) study,[86] the early albumin resuscitation during septic shock (EARSS) study,[87] and the albumin Italian outcome sepsis (ALBIOS) study,[88] none of which found any increase in mortality associated with albumin use when compared with crystalloid fluids. In fact, a recent meta-analysis of EARSS, ALBIOS, and septic patients in SAFE found that the pooled relative risk of death was actually reduced with the use of albumin compared with crystalloid (0.92, 95% CI 0.84–1.0 $P = .046$).[89] One hypothesis as to the beneficial effect of albumin was ascribed to albumin's anti-inflammatory, antioxidant, and scavenging abilities.[90] The clinical use of albumin in acute burn resuscitation is discussed later under timing and dose.

Colloid Timing and Dose

There are 2 general approaches to initiation of colloids. One is to start resuscitation with a colloid as an immediate dedicated strategy. The other is to introduce colloids later in resuscitation as a responsive strategy when actual or projected crystalloid volumes are excessive (**Table 2**).

Table 2
Summary of various strategies for colloid administration during acute burn resuscitation

Early Dedicated	Colloid	Timing	Dose	Effects of Colloid
Slater Formula[25]	FFP	Immediately	75 mL/kg/24 h titrated to UOP (with 2000 mL LR/24 h)	Reduced resuscitation volumes, edema/weight gain, and IAP, improved BD clearance
Haifa Formula[24,77]	Plasma	Immediately	1.5 mL/kg/%TBSA burn/24 h (with 1.0 mL/kg/%TBSA burn/24 h)	No controlled studies
Recinos et al,[84] 1975	Albumin	Immediately	2.3% albumin in LR titrated to 30–50 mL/h UOP	Reduced resuscitation volume, trend to higher UOP
Jelenko et al,[85] 1979	Albumin	Immediately	1.25% albumin in 480 mOsm/L HLS titrated to UOP 30–50 mL/h and MAP 60–110 mm Hg	Reduced resuscitation volume, weight gain, and increased restoration of plasma volume
Goodwin et al,[90] 1983	Albumin	Immediately	2.5% albumin in LR titrated to UOP 30–50 mL/h	Reduced resuscitation volume, increased cardiac performance between 12 and 24 h, increased lung water first PB week
Cooper et al,[96] 2006	Albumin	Immediately	2 mL/kg/%TBSA burn/24 h of 5% albumin with 2 mL/kg/%TBSA burn/24 h of LR	Trend to less resuscitation volume, no effect on MOD, ICU LOS, DurVent

Later Responsive	Colloid	Timing + Indication	Dose	Effects of Colloid
Cochran et al,[35] 2007	Albumin	>12 h PB if CXTL rate ≥ twice Parkland for 2 consecutive hours	5% albumin at 1/3 previous CXTL rate and LR at 2/3 previous CXTL rate (1:2 colloid to CXTL)	Associated mortality reduction (0.27, 95% CI: 0.07–0.97)
Ennis et al,[36] 2008	Albumin	>12–18 h if projected 24 h volume is >6 mL/kg/%TBSA burn	Not described	Reduced composite endpoint of ACS + death
Park et al,[38] 2012	Albumin	>12 h if projected 24 h volume is ≥6 mL/kg/%TBSA burn	5% albumin at previous CXTL rate (CXTL is stopped)	Trend to lower resuscitation volume and decreased DurVent, vasopressor use, and mortality
Dulhunty et al,[37] 2008	Albumin	>8 h as bolus for hypotension (MAP <60 mm Hg) or oliguria (UOP <.5 mL/kg/h)	Not described	Reduced risk of extremity compartment syndrome (0.06, 95% CI: 0.007–0.49)

Abbreviations: ACS, abdominal compartment syndrome; BD, base deficit; CXTL, crystalloid; DurVent, duration of mechanical ventilation; IAP, intra-abdominal pressure; ICU LOS, intensive care unit length of stay; MAP, mean arterial pressure; MOD, multiple organ dysfunction; PB, post burn; UOP, urine output.

Immediate dedicated colloid use

The aforementioned Slater and Haifa Formulas are examples of immediate dedicated colloid provision, using plasma (see **Table 2**). HA solutions have also been used in an immediate dedicated fashion and have been studied in 4 important controlled trials, beginning with Recinos and colleagues,[84] who compared resuscitation with 25 g of albumin in LR (a 2.3% solution) to LR alone among 29 burned children and adults. Limitations of this study included an unclear randomization technique, unspecified blinding, possible baseline differences between intervention and control, and un-identified fluid resuscitation protocol in each study arm. Subjects resuscitated with HA received significantly less fluid than those given LR alone (3.4 mL/kg/%TBSA burn/24 hours vs 5.2 mL/kg/%TBSA burn/24 hours, $P = .001$ in children; and 2.0 mL/kg/%TBSA burn/24 hours vs 2.9 mL/kg/%TBSA burn/24 hours in adults, $P = .001$). Urine output tended to be higher in subjects resuscitated with HA, and there was one case of acute renal failure in the LR group and none in the albumin group.

Jelenko and colleagues[85] compared resuscitation with LR, hypertonic lactated saline (HLS-480 mOsm/L), and HLS+1.25% HA (HL-A) among 19 adults with burns 20% or greater TBSA in a prospective randomized study. The method of randomization was not disclosed. The first 24-hour fluid requirements were significantly lower in the HL-A group (2 mL/kg/%TBSA burn) than in either the HLS (3 mL/kg/%TBSA burn) or the LR group (5.7 mL/kg/%TBSA burn), and subjects in the LR group gained 8 times more weight from edema than from the HL-A group by 72 hours. Restoration of plasma volume occurred significantly sooner in the HL-A subjects than in the other 2 groups. Generalization of these findings is impossible because the study did not assess HA alone and the combination of HA with HLS is not a currently used resuscitation strategy.

Goodwin and colleagues[90] conducted what is probably the most important RCT of albumin versus crystalloid in which 79 severely burned adults without inhalation injury were randomized to either LR or 2.5% HA in LR. Albumin-resuscitated patients required significantly less fluid than the crystalloid-treated patients (2.98 mL/kg/% TBSA burn/24 hours vs 3.81 mL/kg/%TBSA burn/24 hours, $P<.01$). In 29 subjects (15 albumin and 14 crystalloid with no significant differences in 24-hour resuscitation volumes), left ventricular function was assessed. Contractility was similar between the 2 groups but the end-diastolic volume and stroke index, which were depressed in both groups between 0 and 12 hours after burn, were restored to significantly higher levels between 12 and 24 hours in the albumin group as compared with the crystalloid group. This difference had disappeared by 48 hours.

The most controversial and still debated findings from this study had to do with lung water, which remained unchanged in the crystalloid group but which had increased significantly in the albumin-treated subjects by the end of the first week. The investigators concluded that the early administered albumin had gained access to the lung interstitium because of the acute capillary leak and had then subsequently exerted an osmotic force leading to fluid retention in the lung interstitium.

The notion that immediate use of colloid promoted lung edema remained as one of the lasting conclusions of this study and probably contributed to the decline in use of colloids in the first 24 hours that was seen in the 1970s (in addition to Moyer's emphasis on replenishment of extravascular salt and water deficiency with balanced salt solutions[12] and Pruitt's concern that colloids appeared to be no better than crystalloids as volume expanders in the early after-burn period[15]).

However, the conclusion of Goodwin and colleagues on colloid and lung water should be carefully scrutinized. First, their proposed mechanism is not supported by numerous animal studies that have shown maintenance of normal protein sieving and capillary permeability in the lung after burn,[49–51] or by studies that have not found meaningful differences in lung water related to burn resuscitation with crystalloid or albumin.[57,91] Also, animal studies[58] and human studies[92–94] have found that early accumulation of extravascular lung water related to cutaneous burn injury is relatively uncommon. Second, many factors can potentially affect lung edema and were not accounted for in Goodwin's study, including the amount of colloid and free water administered after 24 hours, serum protein levels over the first after burn week, the incidence of sepsis, and differences in mechanical ventilation techniques, especially the amount of positive end-expiratory pressure.[95] Therefore, whether immediate albumin administration is connected to increased lung interstitial fluid development remains unknown.

Last, Cooper and colleagues[96] compared LR to LR plus 5% HA in 42 adults with burns 20% or greater TBSA. Assigned study fluid (5% HA) and control fluid (LR) were also administered after the resuscitation phase up to the time of wound closure. No differences in the primary outcome measure of multiple organ dysfunction or secondary outcomes, including 28-day mortality, duration of mechanical ventilation, and length of intensive care unit stay, were observed. There was a statistically insignificant trend toward a smaller volume of administered study fluid (HA or LR) in the albumin group (3355 mL, 95% CI: 2588–9183 vs 6178 mL, 95% CI: 3435–9481, $P = .42$). This study was halted at 42 subjects of a planned 90 because of slow enrollment.

These studies were small and inadequately powered individually to measure survival differences. However, recent meta-analysis identified that among these 4 randomized trials there was no overall effect of albumin use on mortality (odds ratio [OR] 1.41, 95% CI: 0.27–7.35).[97]

Later responsive use of colloids

Colloids, most notably HA, have also been administered during acute burn resuscitation to "rescue" patients in situations where excessive crystalloid fluid volumes are being given or where resuscitation has become "difficult."[35–38] In the studies' summaries in **Table 2**, albumin was initiated after 12 hours in most of the studies[35,36,38] and after 8 hours in one study.[37] The indications for starting albumin were predominantly based on actual or projected crystalloid volumes exceeding the Parkland formula by 50% to 100%,[35,36,38] but in one study, albumin was used as a "bolus fluid" for oliguria (<0.5 mL/kg/h) or hypotension (mean arterial pressure <60 mm Hg).[37]

When reported, the dose of albumin varied between providing one-third to 100% of the previous crystalloid hourly rate as albumin.[35,38] This approach to albumin use was generally associated with improvements in outcome, including increased survival, shorter duration of mechanical ventilation, and reduced limb compartment syndrome. A volume-sparing effect of albumin is difficult to ascertain in most of these studies because albumin was being given to reduce excessive resuscitation volumes. However, a study by Lawrence and colleagues[98] demonstrated a profound effect of albumin when used in this fashion as a volume-sparing agent. Furthermore, when the meta-analysis by Navickis and colleagues[97] considered prospective and retrospective studies that reported extremity compartment syndrome,[36–38,85,96] albumin use was associated with an 81% relative decrease in the risk of this complication (pooled OR 0.19, 95% CI: 0.07–0.50, $P<.001$).[97]

Clinical colloid resuscitation—key points

- HES, dextran, and gelatins are effective volume expanders, but current safety concerns prevent use or recommendation of these colloids in burn resuscitation.

- FFP is an effective volume-sparing colloid for burn resuscitation, but its benefits must be weighed against its cost and potential for virus transmission and induction of TRALI.

- Albumin has demonstrated volume-sparing effects when used immediately or later in burn resuscitation, possibly leading to improved outcome. It is not known if albumin increases lung extravascular water.

SUMMARY

Colloids have been used in varying capacities throughout the history of formula-based burn resuscitation. There is sound experimental evidence that demonstrates colloids' ability to improve intravascular colloid osmotic pressure, expand intravascular volume, reduce resuscitation requirements, and limit edema in unburned tissue following a major burn. FFP appears to be a useful and effective immediate burn resuscitation fluid, but its benefits must be weighed against its costs and risks of viral transmission and acute lung injury. Albumin, in contrast, is less expensive and safer and has demonstrated ability to reduce resuscitation requirements and possibly limit edema-related morbidity. Unquestionably, a large modern prospective evaluation of albumin versus crystalloid is needed.

REFERENCES

1. Pruitt BA. Fluid resuscitation. J Trauma 1981;21(Suppl 8):667–8.
2. Greenhalgh DG. Burn resuscitation. J Burn Care Res 2007;28:555–65.
3. Pham TN, Cancio LG, Gibran NS. American Burn Association practice guidelines burn shock resuscitation. J Burn Care Res 2008;29:257–66.
4. Greenhalgh DG. Burn resuscitation: the results of the ISBI/ABA survey. Burns 2010;36:176–82.
5. Cope O, Moore FD. The redistribution of body water and the fluid therapy of the burned patient. Ann Surg 1947;126:1013(footnote).
6. Cope O, Moore FD. The redistribution of body water and the fluid therapy of the burned patient. Ann Surg 1947;126:1010–45.
7. Moore FD. The body-weight burn budget. Surg Clin North Am 1970;50:1249–65.
8. Evans EI, Purnell OJ, Robinett PW, et al. Fluid and electrolyte requirements in severe burns. J Trauma 1952;135:804–15.
9. Fox CL, Baer H. Redistribution of potassium sodium and water in burns and trauma and its relation to the phenomenon of shock. Am J Physiol 1947;151: 155–67.
10. Rosenthal SM. Experimental chemotherapy of burns and shock III: effects of systemic therapy on early mortality. Publ Health Rep 1943;58:513–22.
11. Reiss E, Stirman JA, Artz CP, et al. Fluid and electrolyte balance in burns. JAMA 1953;152:1309–13.
12. Moyer CA, Margraf HW, Monafo WW. Burn shock and extravascular sodium deficiency—treatment with Ringer's solution with lactate. Arch Surg 1965;90: 799–810.
13. Baxter CR, Shires T. Physiologic response to crystalloid resuscitation of severe burns. Ann N Y Acad Sci 1968;150:874–94.

14. Baxter CR. Fluid volume and electrolyte changes of the early post burn period. Clin Plast Surg 1974;1:693–709.
15. Pruitt BA Jr, Mason AD, Moncrief JA. Hemodynamic changes in the early post burn patient: the influence of fluid administration and of a vasodilator (hydralazine). J Trauma 1971;11:36–46.
16. Pruitt BA Jr. Fluid resuscitation for the extensively burned patient. J Trauma 1981; 21(Suppl 8):690–2.
17. Pruitt BA Jr. Advances in fluid therapy and the early care of the burn patient. World J Surg 1978;2:139–50.
18. Baxter CR, Marvin J, Curreri PW. Fluid and electrolyte therapy of burn shock. Heart Lung 1973;2:707–13.
19. Janeway CA, Gibson ST, Woodruff LM, et al. Chemical, clinical, and immunological studies on the products of human plasma fractionation VII: concentrated human albumin solution. J Clin Invest 1944;23:465–90.
20. Herndon DN, Barrow RE, Linares HA, et al. Inhalation injury in burned patients: effects and treatment. Burns 1988;14:349–56.
21. Darling GE, Kerestechi MA, Ibanez, et al. Pulmonary complications in inhalation injuries with associated cutaneous burns. J Trauma 1996;40:83–9.
22. Shimazaki S, Yukioka T, Matuda H. Fluid distribution and pulmonary dysfunction following burn shock. J Trauma 1991;31:623–8.
23. Muir I. The use of the Mount Vernon formula in the treatment of burn shock. Intensive Care Med 1981;7:49–53.
24. Ullmann Y, Kremer R, Ramon Y, et al. Evaluation of the validity of the Haifa formula for fluid resuscitation in burn patients at the Rambam Medical Centre. Ann Burns Fire Disasters 2000;13:1–10.
25. Du G, Slater H, Goldfarb IW. Influences of different resuscitation regimens on acute early weight gain in extensively burned patients. Burns 1991;17:147–50.
26. Wharton SM, Khanna A. Current attitudes to burns resuscitation in the UK. Burns 2001;27:183–4.
27. Cochrane Injuries Group. Human albumin administration in critically ill patients: systematic review of randomized controlled trials. BMJ 1998;317:235–40.
28. Offringa M. Excess mortality after human albumin ad-ministration in critically ill patients. Clinical and pathophysiological evidence suggests albumin is harmful. BMJ 1998;317:223–4.
29. Cole RP. The UK albumin debate. Burns 1999;25:565–8.
30. Pruitt BA Jr. Protection from excessive resuscitation: "pushing the pendulum back". J Trauma 2000;49:567–8.
31. Cartotto R, Innes M, Musgrave MA, et al. How well does the Parkland formula estimate actual fluid resuscitation volumes? J Burn Care Rehabil 2002;23:258–65.
32. Cancio LC, Chávez S, Alvarado-Ortega M, et al. Predicting increased fluid requirements during the resuscitation of thermally injured patients. J Trauma 2004;56:404–13 [discussion: 413–4].
33. Grady JJ, Mitchell CE, Salinas J, et al. Meta-analysis of fluid requirements for burn injury. J Burn Care Res 2010;31:S97.
34. Saffle JR. The phenomenon of "fluid creep" in acute burn resuscitation. J Burn Care Res 2007;28:382–95.
35. Cochran A, Morris SE, Edelman LS, et al. Burn patient characteristics and outcomes following resuscitation with albumin. Burns 2007;33:25–30.
36. Ennis JL, Chung KK, Renz EM, et al. Joint theater trauma system implementation of burn resuscitation guidelines improves outcomes in severely burned military casualties. J Trauma 2008;64(2 Suppl):S146–51 [discussion: S151–2].

37. Dulhunty JM, Boots RJ, Rudd MJ, et al. Increased fluid resuscitation can lead to adverse outcomes in major burn injured patients, but low mortality is achievable. Burns 2008;34:1090–7.
38. Park SH, Hemmila MR, Wahl W. Early albumin use improves mortality in difficult to resuscitate patients. J Trauma Acute Care Surg 2012;73:1294–7.
39. Starling EH. On the absorption of fluids from the connective tissue spaces. J Physiol 1896;19:312–26.
40. Chappell D, Jacob M, Hofmann-Kiefer K, et al. A rational approach to perioperative fluid management. Anesthesiology 2008;109:723–40.
41. Demling RH. The burn edema process: current concepts. J Burn Care Rehabil 2005;26:207–27.
42. Landis EM. Heteroporosity of the capillary wall as indicated by cinematographic analysis of the passage of dyes. Ann N Y Acad Sci 1964;16:765–73.
43. Levick JR, Michel CC. Microvascular fluid exchange and the revised Starling Principle. Cardiovasc Res 2010;87:198–210.
44. Cope O, Graham JB, Moore FD, et al. The nature of the shift of plasma protein to the extravascular space following thermal injury. Ann Surg 1948;128:1041–55.
45. Netsky MG, Leiter SS. Capillary permeability to horse proteins in burn shock. Am J Physiol 1943;140:1–7.
46. Arturson G. Microvascular permeability to macromolecules in thermal injury. Acta Physiol Scand Suppl 1979;463:111–22.
47. Nanney LB. Changes in the microvasculature of skin subjected to thermal injury. Burns 1982;8:321–7.
48. Pitt RM, Parker JC, Jurkovich GJ, et al. Analysis of altered capillary pressure and permeability after thermal injury. J Surg Res 1987;42:693–702.
49. Demling RH, Smith M, Bodai B, et al. Comparison of post-burn capillary permeability in soft tissue and lung. J Burn Care Rehabil 1981;15:86–92.
50. Demling RH, Kramer GC, Gunther R, et al. Effect of nonprotein colloid on post-burn edema formation in soft tissues and lung. Surgery 1984;95:593–602.
51. Harms BA, Bodai BI, Kramer GC, et al. Microvascular fluid and protein flux in pulmonary and systemic circulations after thermal injury. Microvasc Res 1982;23:77–86.
52. Bert J, Gyenge C, Bowen B, et al. Fluid resuscitation following a burn injury: implications of a mathematical model of microvascular exchange. Burns 1997;23:93–105.
53. Demling RH, Kramer G, Harms B. Role of thermal in-jury-induced hypoproteinemia on fluid flux and protein permeability in burned and nonburned tissue. Surgery 1984;95:136–44.
54. Guha SC, Kinsky MP, Button B, et al. Burn resuscitation: crystalloid versus colloid versus hypertonic saline hyperoncotic colloid in sheep. Crit Care Med 1996;24:1849–57.
55. Vlachou E, Moieman NS. Microalbuminemia: a marker of endothelial dysfunction in thermal injury. Burns 2006;32:1009–16.
56. Onarheim H, Reed RK. Thermal skin injury: effect of fluid therapy on the transcapillary colloid osmotic gradient. J Surg Res 1991;50:272–8.
57. Mehrkens HH, Ahnefeld FW. Volume and fluid replacement in the early post burn period: an animal experimental study. Burns 1979;5:113–5.
58. Asch MJ, Feldman RJ, Walker HL, et al. Systemic and pulmonary hemodynamic changes accompanying thermal in-jury. Ann Surg 1973;178:218–21.
59. Haase N, Perner A. Hydroxyethyl starch for resuscitation. Curr Opin Crit Care 2013;19:321–5.

60. Waters LM, Christenson MA, Sato RM. Hetastarch: an alternative colloid in burn shock management. J Burn Care Rehabil 1989;10:11–5.
61. Waxman K, Holness R, Tominaga G, et al. Hemodynamic and oxygen transport effects of pentastarch in burn resuscitation. Ann Surg 1989;209:341–5.
62. Vlachou E, Gosling P, Moieman NS. Hydroxyethylstarch supplementation in burn resuscitation—a prospective randomized controlled trial. Burns 2010;36:984–91.
63. Béchir M, Puhan MA, Fasshauer M, et al. Early fluid resuscitation with hydroxyethyl starch 130/0.4 (6%) in severe burn injury: a randomized controlled double-blind trial. Crit Care 2013;17:R299.
64. Myburgh JA, Finfer S, Bellomo R, et al. Hydroxyethyl starch or saline for fluid resuscitation in intensive care. N Engl J Med 2012;367:1901–11.
65. Perner A, Haase N, Guttormsen AB, et al. Hydroxyethyl starch 130/0.42 versus Ringer's acetate in severe sepsis. N Engl J Med 2012;367:124–34.
66. Guidet B, Martinet O, Boulain T, et al. Assessment of hemodynamic efficacy and safety of fluid replacement in patients with severe sepsis: the CRYSTMAS study. Crit Care 2012;16:R94.
67. Medicines and Healthcare Products Regulatory Agency. Class 2 drug alert (action within 48 hours): hydroxyethyl starch (HES) products—B Braun Melsungen AG and Fresenius Kabi Limited. Available at: http://www.mhra.gov.uk/Publications/Safetywarnings/DrugAlerts/CON287025. Accessed July 4, 2013.
68. Food and Drug Administration. FDA safety communication: boxed warning on increased mortality and severe renal injury, and additional warning on risk of bleeding, for use of hydroxyethyl starch solutions in some settings. Available at: http://www.fda.gov/BiologicsBloodVaccines/.../ucm358271.htm.
69. Thomas-Rueddell DO, Vlasakov V, Reinhart K, et al. Safety of gelatins for volume resuscitation—a systematic review and meta-analysis. Intensive Care Med 2012;38:1134–42.
70. Elgjo GI, Poli de Figueiredo LF, Schenarts PJ, et al. Hypertonic saline dextran produces early (8-12 hrs) fluid sparing in burn resuscitation: a 24-hr prospective, double-blind study in sheep. Crit Care Med 2000;28(1):163–71.
71. Nascimento B, Callum J, Rubenfeld G, et al. Clinical review: fresh frozen plasma in massive bleeding—more questions than answers. Crit Care 2010;14:201–10.
72. Higgins S, Fowler R, Callum J, et al. Transfusion-related acute lung injury in patients with burns. J Burn Care Res 2007;28(1):56–64.
73. O'Mara MS, Slater H, Goldfarb IW, et al. A prospective, randomized evaluation of intra-abdominal pressures with crystalloid and colloid resuscitation in burn patients. J Trauma 2005;58:1011–8.
74. Choi J, Cooper A, Gomez M, et al. The 2000 Moyer Award: the relevance of base deficits after burn injuries. J Burn Care Rehabil 2000;21(6):499–505.
75. Aharoni A, Abramovici D, Weinberger M, et al. Burn resuscitation with a low volume plasma regimen—analysis of mortality. Burns 1989;15:230–2.
76. Aharoni A, Moscona R, Kremerman S, et al. Pulmonary complications in burn patients resuscitated with low volume colloid solution. Burns 1989;15:281–4.
77. Fodor L, Fodor A, Ramon Y, et al. Controversies in fluid resuscitation for burn management: literature review and our experience. Injury 2006;37:374–9.
78. Nicholson JP, Wolmarans MR, Park GR. The role of albumin in critical illness. Br J Anaesth 2000;85:599–610.
79. Fanali G, di Masi A, Trezza V, et al. Human serum albumin: from bench to bedside. Mol Aspects Med 2012;33:209–90.
80. Laub R, Strengers P. Parvoviruses and blood products. Pathol Biol 2002;50:339–48.

81. Food and Drug Administration. Guidance for industry: revised preventive measures to reduce the possible risk of transmission of Creutzfeldt-Jakob disease and variant Creutzfeldt-Jakob disease by blood and blood products. 2012. Available at: http://www.fda.gov/downloads/biologicsbloodvaccines/guidance complianceregulatoryinformation/guidances/blood/ucm307137.pdf. Accessed August 3, 2014.

82. Margarson MP, Soni NC. Changes in serum albumin concentration and volume expanding effects following a bolus of albumin 20% in septic patients. Br J Anaesth 2004;92:821–6.

83. Greenhalgh DG, Housinger TA, Kagan RJ, et al. Maintenance of serum albumin levels in pediatric burn patients: a prospective, randomized trial. J Trauma 1995;39:67–73 [discussion: 73–4].

84. Recinos PR, Hartford CA, Ziffren SE. Fluid resuscitation of burn patients comparing a crystalloid with a colloid containing solution: a prospective study. J Iowa Med Soc 1975;65:426–32.

85. Jelenko C 3rd, Williams JB, Wheeler ML, et al. Studies in shock and resuscitation, I: use of a hypertonic, albumin-containing, fluid demand regimen (HALFD) in resuscitation. Crit Care Med 1979;7:157–67.

86. Finfer S, Bellomo R, Boyce N. A comparison of albumin and saline for fluid resuscitation in the intensive care unit. N Engl J Med 2004;350:2247–56.

87. Charpentier J, Mira JP, EARSS Study Group. Efficacy and tolerance of hyperoncotic albumin administration in septic shock patients: the EARSS Study. Intensive Care Med 2011;37(Suppl 1):S115.

88. Caironi P, Tognoni G, Masson S, et al. Albumin replacement in patients with severe sepsis or septic shock. N Engl J Med 2014;370:1412–21.

89. Wieddermann CJ, Joannidid M. Albumin replacement in severe sepsis or septic shock. N Engl J Med 2014;371:83–4.

90. Goodwin CW, Dorethy J, Lam V, et al. Randomized trial of efficacy of crystalloid and colloid resuscitation on hemodynamic response and lung water following thermal injury. Ann Surg 1983;197:520–31.

91. Holleman JH, Gabel JC, Hardy JD. Pulmonary effects of intravenous fluid therapy in burn resuscitation. Surg Gynecol Obstet 1978;147:161–6.

92. Tranbaugh RF, Lewis FR, Christensen JM, et al. Lung water changes after thermal injury. The effects of crystalloid resuscitation and sepsis. Ann Surg 1980;192:479–90.

93. Holm C, Tegeler J, Mayr M, et al. Effect of crystalloid resuscitation and inhalation injury on extravascular lung water: clinical implications. Chest 2002;121:1956–62.

94. Tranbaugh RF, Elings VB, Christensen JM, et al. Effect of inhalation injury on lung water accumulation. J Trauma 1983;23:597–604.

95. Maybauer DM, Talke PO, Westphal M, et al. Positive end-expiratory pressure ventilation increases extravascular lung water due to a decrease in lung lymph flow. Anaesth Intensive Care 2006;34:329–33.

96. Cooper AB, Cohn SM, Zhang HS, et al. Five percent albumin for adult burn shock resuscitation: lack of effect on daily multiple organ dysfunction score. Transfusion 2006;46:80–9.

97. Navickis RJ, Greenhalgh DG, Wilkes MM. Albumin in burn shock resuscitation: a meta-analysis of controlled clinical studies. J Burn Care Res 2016;37(3):e268–78.

98. Lawrence A, Faraklas I, Watkins H, et al. Colloid administration normalizes resuscitation ratio and ameliorates "fluid creep". J Burn Care Res 2010;31:40–7.

Monitoring End Points of Burn Resuscitation

Daniel M. Caruso, MD*, Marc R. Matthews, MD

KEYWORDS

- Burn resuscitation • End points • Burn shock • End points of resuscitation

KEY POINTS

- Burn care is best provided in a regional burn center that has the expertise and experience in caring for a unique population of critically ill patients.
- Although burn resuscitation is monitored and administered using the methodology as seen in medical/surgical intensive care settings, special consideration for excessive edema formation, metabolic derangements and frequent operative interventions must be considered.
- End points of burn resuscitation must be able to consider these factors and provide reliable starting and stopping points.

INTRODUCTION
Shock and Burn Shock

Described in the nineteenth century by Gross,[1] shock was believed to be a "manifestation of the crude unhinging of the machinery of life." Years later, shock was noted by Blalock[2] to be "a peripheral circulatory failure, resulting from a discrepancy in the size of the vascular bed and the volume of the intravascular fluid." In present day, the 2006 International Consensus Conference and American College of Surgeons Advanced Trauma Life Support defined shock by using degrees of derangements in physiologic parameters, such as heart rate, urine output, and blood pressure.[3] These efforts yielded the current definition of shock as "an abnormality of the circulatory system that results in inadequate organ perfusion and tissue oxygenation"; failure of a person's oxygen supply to meet their tissue metabolic demands.[4]

Burn shock is the significant loss of fluids described as a combination of hypovolemic and distributive shock.[5–10] Although shock states often require significant fluid administration, burn resuscitation often requires supertherapeutic fluid administration to maintain adequate perfusion and ultimately restore fluid balance. Unfortunately, fluid administration in the burn shock state is easier said than done. Systemic capillary

Disclosure Statement: The authors have nothing to disclose.
Department of Surgery, The Arizona Burn Center, 2601 East Roosevelt, Phoenix, AZ 85008, USA
* Corresponding author.
E-mail address: Daniel_Caruso@dmgaz.org

leak from the microcirculation causes protein (decreasing osmotic pressure) and fluid loss from the vascular system.[5,9,11,12] Excessive fluid movement occurs into the interstitium resulting in a decrease in plasma volume, hemoconcentration, global edema, low urine output, and increasing systemic vascular resistance.[7,13] Coupled with the grave fluid losses is the release of tumor necrosis factor-α, which acts directly on the cardiac myocardium to decrease contractility and cardiac output (CO).[7,14,15] Next, edema formation, although stated to be maximal at 24 hours post burn injury, often continues for 48 to 72 hours resulting in tissue hypoxia, increased tissue pressure, and possible compartment syndromes.[5,9,11] To restore the plasma volume the extracellular space must be expanded but in doing so may actually worsen the edema.[9,16,17]

Goals of Burn Resuscitation and Monitoring

Resuscitation is the restoration of a body's normal physiology, primarily at the cellular level. Although normal physiologic values may be obtained, persistent hypoxemia, anaerobic acidosis, and lactic acidosis may still be present. Thus, many burn practitioners have noted that the ideal burn resuscitation protocol would prevent rather than treat burn shock.[18–20] These same clinicians argue that resuscitation of burn shock cannot achieve complete normalization of physiologic parameters because of the burn injury, subsequent operative treatment, and ongoing cellular and hormonal responses. Among burn physicians there is considerable variability in determining the type and amount of fluids to be administered and how to monitor and ultimately cease resuscitation efforts. Thus burn resuscitation is an area of clinical practice driven primarily by local custom of treating burn units than by evidence-based medicine.[21] More sophisticated physiologic markers, also known as end points of resuscitation, have been sought to better guide resuscitative efforts in patients undergoing shock.

END POINTS OF BURN RESUSCITATION
First-Line Monitoring

Even though burn physicians are aware of the limitations of monitoring resuscitation using heart rate and urine output, Latenser[21] noted that these parameters are still the primary modalities, although their use in patients with large burns is not supported by data. Most burn physicians use the standard that a pulse rate less than 110 beats/min in adults usually indicates adequate volume, with rates greater than 120 beats/min usually indicating hypovolemia. Narrowed pulse pressure provides an earlier indication of shock than systolic blood pressure alone.[5] Furthermore, noninvasive blood pressure measurements by cuff are rendered inaccurate because of the interference of tissue edema.[12] Therefore, arterial catheter placement is recommended. However restoration of blood pressure to the normal range, although the most common method of resuscitation, demonstrates great variability in terms of the accuracy of systolic and diastolic pressures. Most often, clinicians rely on mean arterial blood pressure (MAP) has a more accurate blood pressure measurement.

When MAP is normalized it is termed an end point of resuscitation, all be it controversial. In 2001, Rivers and colleagues[22] reported the substantial benefits of using MAP in early goal-directed therapy. They demonstrated that a significant mortality decrease was possible in patients with sepsis treated with an algorithm including MAP, central venous pressure (CVP), and mixed venous oxygen saturation (SvO₂). However, Donnino and colleagues[23] later reported that despite normalization of MAP, a significant number of patients were still exhibiting signs of global hypoxia revealed by lactic acidosis. Despite controversies related to this study, the 2012 Surviving Sepsis Guidelines has recommended a goal MAP of 65 or higher during the first 6 hours of resuscitation in septic shock.[24] It should be noted that MAP of 65 or higher is often used by burn physicians when determining adequate resuscitation.

Urine output is still the most commonly used single basic end point of resuscitation in the burn community. However, Latenser[20,21] also pointed out that reliance on hourly urine output as the sole index of optimum resuscitation sharply contrasts with the lack of clinical studies demonstrating the ideal hourly urine output during resuscitation. Even so, the American Burn Association Practice Guidelines for Burn Shock Resuscitation still recommend a urine output of 0.5 mL/kg/h in adults and 0.5 to 1.0 mL/kg/h in children weighing less than 30 kg.[5,19] If hourly urinary outputs fall below these standards within the first 48 hours postburn, this almost always represents inadequate resuscitation.[16]

In the final analysis, although these basic parameters are useful in determining the end points of resuscitation, the search for better parameters is ongoing. Currently, resuscitation end points are divided into two large groups based on the information that they can provide. Hemodynamic markers are one group, which includes MAP, SvO_2 and central venous oxygen saturation ($ScvO_2$), CVP, and arterial pulse waveform analysis. Moreover, echocardiography and its hemodynamic values can also provide information regarding the hemodynamic status of a patient. The other category are perfusion end points, which include such methods as base deficit (BD), gastric tonometry, near-infrared spectroscopy (NIRS), and lactate, which are useful indicators to determine oxygenation at a cellular level.

HEMODYNAMIC END POINTS OF RESUSCITATION
Goal-Directed Therapy

In the 1990s, several investigators in the critical care arena touted the benefits of goal-directed therapy in which invasive central venous catheters and/or Swan-Ganz catheters were placed and resuscitation was directed based on hemodynamic parameters obtained. In burn, Schiller and Bay[25] used the published concepts of Shoemaker and others to prospectively study patients requiring large-volume resuscitation.[26,27] Patients were first volume loaded (saline and colloid) to cardiac filling pressures of 12 to 15 mm Hg along with normalization of vital signs and a urine output of at least 1 mg/kg/h. Next, cardiac indices were calculated and enhanced using vasopressor agents to achieve target values of a cardiac index greater than 4.1 L/min/m^2, stroke index greater than 40 m/beat/m^2, left ventricular stroke work index greater than 50 g/mm^2, and oxygen consumption greater than 350 mL/min.[26,27] These authors summarized that during a 5-year period using hyperdynamic circulatory end points allowed patients to withstand a greater degree of organ dysfunction and still survive. However, examination of their data reveals no statistical differences between survivors and nonsurvivors in regards to the amount of fluid infused, colloid infused, cardiotonic medications, cardiac index, stroke work, oxygen consumption, vital signs, or urine output. The only statistical significant difference was that pulmonary artery wedge pressures were higher in the nonsurvival group. Although it was indeed possible to achieve supranormal goals, few patients actually improved and most patients had excessive amounts of fluid with increased mortality above expected norms.

These results should not be surprising. Other investigators have used goal-directed therapy in other populations of the critically ill and demonstrated no change in multiorgan failure, mortality, and outcome.[28,29] What was ultimately found is that oxygen parameter is more useful as a sign of survival in a patient rather than as a goal for the patient's resuscitation.

Latenser and others have noted the lack of benefit associated with goal-directed supranormal therapy and the waning enthusiasm for the use of pulmonary artery catheters.[30,31] Even though the most applicable CO-related variable to manipulate in burn patients is preload, these same authors believe that pulmonary artery occlusion pressure and CVP are not good indicators of preload[5,15] because these static pressure-derived values, such as CVP, do not accurately predict a patient's volume status.[16–19] Conversely, such recommendations as the 2012 Surviving Sepsis Campaign Guidelines clearly state that a CVP of 8 to 12 mm Hg is a "recommended physiologic target for resuscitation" during the first 6 hours of septic shock resuscitation.[14] Therefore, in current burn practice most physicians often trend CVP values to determine fluid status. The temptation, however, to normalize filling pressures should be avoided as long as other signs of adequate tissue perfusion exist.[12]

Mixed Venous Oxygen Saturation/Central Venous Oxygen Saturation

The use of end points demonstrating the adequacy of oxygen delivery has not yet found a place in the management of burn shock.[7] SvO_2 gathered by a venous sample from a central line catheter ($ScvO_2$) represents regional venous oxygen saturation as opposed to global saturation. Although $ScvO_2$ tends to be more practical than SvO_2 because no pulmonary artery catheter is needed, the values gained are usually higher by about 7% compared with the values obtained through SvO_2. The greatest differences in values between the two techniques were found primarily in patients with heart failure, sepsis, and cardiogenic shock.[32] Even though the values were different, trends in $ScvO_2$ and in SvO_2 were generally correlated.[32,33] SvO_2 and $ScvO_2$ are related to oxygen balance in the tissues. A low value is an indicator of tissue hypoxia and the need for continued resuscitation. As general markers SvO_2 and $ScvO_2$ lack the ability to provide information regarding regional or microcirculatory perfusion, especially in septic shock, where such conditions as perfusion heterogeneity may lead to closed capillaries with low saturation and open capillaries that are highly saturated.[34,35]

Even so, the use of $ScvO_2$ has been increasingly supported as an indicator of shock in patients, and decreased values have been found in hypovolemic and cardiogenic shock.[36–38] In septic shock, Rivers and colleagues showed that when an $ScvO_2$ goal of greater than 70% was used in "early goal-directed therapy" survival rates increased by 16%. This finding has led to $ScvO_2$ being used ever increasingly as an end point of resuscitation especially in the septic shock state, which is often seen in the critically ill burn patient.[39]

Arterial Waveform Pulse Analysis

Arterial pulse waveform analysis is used to determine stroke volume (SV) by analyzing pulse pressure waveform data gathered from an arterial catheter. CO is then calculated based on the pulse pressure being directly proportional to SV. Pulse pressure variability in relation to SV is affected by positive pressure ventilation and most noted in volume-depleted patients whose right ventricular filling is decreased. Once blood has cycled a few times the left ventricle also experiences a variation in its filling as blood is pumped through the lungs and back again to the heart. This variation in patients with hypovolemia is termed SV variation.[40] SV variation monitoring has proved useful and accurate in predicting patients that are fluid responsive. Investigators have found that when patients with sepsis were mechanically ventilated there were systolic pressure variations of more than 13% and they were highly sensitive to fluid administration.[41,42]

There are several devices that can be used to evaluate the arterial pulse pressure including the Vigileo/FloTrac system (Edwards Lifesciences, Irvine, CA), which uses a software algorithm to analyze arterial waveforms and ultimately determine CO.[43,44] Advances on this technology include the LiDCO Plus system (LiDCO, Cambridge, UK), which is capable of determining SV and CO using a lithium-based dye dilution technique.[45] Another technology is the PiCCO monitor (Pulsion, Munich, Germany), which combines thermodilution with waveform analysis to determine a patient's CO and lung water and cardiac chamber volumes. The downside to this method is that a central arterial and a central venous vessel must be invaded to get accurate readings.[46]

Unfortunately, only a few small-scale trials have been performed using arterial waveform analysis and goal-directed therapy in the resuscitation of patients.[47–49] Although each of these devices have advantages and disadvantages the overwhelming limitation of each waveform system is that in the setting of cardiac arrhythmias, aortic valve regurgitation, and in peripheral vascular disease their validity is greatly reduced. Moreover, waveform analysis is further limited by the necessity of a patient having a respiratory rate of 17 breathes per minute or less. In the critically ill burn patient who often has cardiac and/or respiratory dysfunction and may require nonconventional modes of mechanical ventilation, arterial waveform systems have significant limitations especially during acute resuscitation.

Echocardiography

Echocardiography has become commonplace at the intensive care bedside because of its ease of access and usability. Echocardiography, either transthoracic or transesophageal, allows access to images and information about a patient's cardiac anatomy, assessment of cardiac function, ventricular volume, CO, and ejection fraction.[50] Images are gathered as static and/or dynamic parameters, such as overall volume status, filling pressures, and SV. The measurement of SV in the left ventricle is obtained by using an equation: velocity time interval (VTI) multiplied by the cross-sectional area of the aortic annulus. Changes in VTI correspond to changes in SV, which is an important resuscitation end point.[51,52] A study performed by Monnet and colleagues[53] found that hypovolemia and fluid responsiveness could be detected in mechanically ventilated patients when VTI was being monitored. Feissel and colleagues also found that patients in septic shock during fluid resuscitation that were mechanically ventilated demonstrated changes in VTI that accurately predicted increases in CO.[54] Echocardiography can also be used to analyze the size of the inferior vena cava (IVC) allowing clinicians to assess preload and volume responsiveness. A study by Ferrada and colleagues[55] found that patients who were administered a fluid bolus when their IVC was determined to be less than 2 cm by a transthoracic echocardiogram then had an increase in their IVC diameter to greater than 2 cm, leading to a 97% resolution of hypotension. When used in the monitoring of mechanically ventilated patients two studies found that echocardiography was able to provide data showing that fluid responsiveness is predictable by monitoring respiratory variations in IVC diameter.[55,56]

A major criticisms of echocardiography is that accuracy is based on proficiency of the user. Although some of the information obtained may only require minimal training, such as the ability to determine IVC diameter, analysis of the dynamic parameters requires advanced training. For example, the clinician must be able to successfully determination respiratory changes in SV based on VTI.[54] Even so, the use of bedside echocardiography is not only beneficial in the evaluation and resuscitation of patients who are in shock but its overall noninvasive nature makes it ideal. Because few studies exist examining the use of echocardiography in burn resuscitation, more investigation is needed.[57]

PERFUSION MARKERS
Lactate

Lactate, a by-product of glucose, is formed as glucose is metabolized in glycolysis to pyruvate, which is either converted into ATP or lactate. Pyruvate can only be turned into ATP when oxygen is present. In the setting of hypoxia and/or hypoperfusion, the deficit of oxygen supply causes pyruvate not to be converted into ATP (via mitochondria), but instead to be converted directly into lactate.[58] Lactate when used as an end point of resuscitation has demonstrated a strong correlation to mortality. In one study of 95 critically ill patients, normalizing lactate levels quickly improved overall mortality. If lactate was normalized in less than 24 hours, patients had 3.9% mortality versus normalization at 24 to 48 hours yielding a mortality rate of 13.3%. At 49 to 98 hours patients suffered a mortality rate of 42.5%.[58] Another staggering statistic is when a patient was unable to normalize their lactate level they faced a mortality rate of approximately 100%.

Lactate clearance has become an integral part of many goal-directed resuscitation protocols especially when the lactate levels remain elevated. A trial by Jones and colleagues[59] compared the effectiveness of resuscitation using lactate clearance with resuscitation using $ScvO_2$. Patients who cleared lactate effectively had a mortality rate that was 6% lower than the group resuscitated to a $ScvO_2$. In another study, patients resuscitated via lactate levels had a morality rate of 10% versus those resuscitated via unguided parameters who demonstrated mortality rates of 33.9% to 43.5%.[60] The group resuscitated via lactate levels also recovered quicker, where removed from support systems sooner, and were discharged from the intensive care setting in a shorter time span then the others who were left unguided.[58]

Level of lactate in the blood is a balance between production and removal, filtered by the liver and kidneys.[61,62] If either liver or kidney dysfunction exists, the excretion of lactate is blunted, even if the patient has no signs of hypoperfusion, sepsis, and/or shock. Furthermore, lactate clearance can be unresponsive because of the presence of sepsis or mesenteric ischemia. Thus, some authors argue that although lactate is a strong predictor of mortality, it is not clear how serum lactate can be used as a resuscitation end point, especially in the burn population.[5,12,63]

Base Deficit

BD is a marker for lactic acidosis and anaerobic metabolism. Common clinical values are a range of −3 to +3 mmol, the negative values demonstrating lactic acidosis. In trauma patients, BD is an accurate measure of a patient's hypoperfusion. In a study by Rutherford and colleagues,[64] BD was tested to determine what BD level would be a predictor of mortality. In patients younger than age 55 a BD of −15 mmol within a 24-hour period postinjury was a significant marker of mortality. In patients older than 55 years of age a BD value of −8 mmol was a significant sign of mortality; older patients have less tolerance of the acidotic state.[64] In another study, Mutschler and colleagues[65] showed that BD could be organized into classes that would predict mortality. Four categories of BD levels were developed: less than 2 mmol/dL (class 1), 2 to 6 mmol/dL (class 2), 6 to 10 mmol/dL (class 3), and greater than 10 mmol/dL (class 4). Patients in the class 3 and 4 groups had significantly higher rates of mortality and risk of coagulopathy, and were more prone to transfusion therapy, hypovolemic shock, acute respiratory distress syndrome, and renal failure compared with those in groups 1 or 2.[66,67]

Although BD might be a good predictor of survivability, its use as a marker of perfusion is limited. BD levels can be significantly affected by hypothermia or simply the administration of sodium bicarbonate and/or tris-hydroxymethyl aminomethane. Alcohol, in large quantities, can have a profound effect on BD levels, and can be altered by carbon dioxide (CO_2) retention, renal failure, and diabetic ketoacidosis.[68,69] All of this makes the use of BD unreliable in the patient undergoing resuscitative efforts.[70,71]

In burn patients, Latenser points out that although lactate and BD are resuscitation markers that act as independent variables, there is a low correlation between urinary output, MAP, serum lactate, and BD. Serum lactate trends provide greater information regarding the homeostatic status but determinations of BD do not demonstrate the same predictive power.[21,72,73] Overall, the effect of specific correction of the BD during fluid resuscitation is unknown.[21] Although trauma studies have shown that if lactate and BD are corrected quickly this can significantly lower mortality rates,[64] there are still insufficient data to make recommendations on the use of BD or lactate as resuscitation guidelines during burn resuscitation or as independent predictors of outcome in patients with large burns.[5,12,21]

Near-Infrared Spectroscopy

NIRS is a noninvasive procedure that measures the regional oxidation of the tissue. Using fiberoptic light, NIRS analyzes a patient's chromophomes to determine their oxygen concentration (via DO_2 measurements) at a selected tissue area.[74] Most NIRS machines use the palmar thumb tissue and its muscle directly beneath (often limited in its edema formation during sepsis/shock) as the ideal area for selected tissue oxygen measurement (StO_2). Unfortunately, although NIRS is appealing because of its noninvasiveness it is not completely reliable as an indicator of oxygenation. In some studies, StO_2 levels have been found not to change in the critically ill state compared with healthy patients.[75–77]

A study of nonshock volunteers was compared with trauma patients on a scale that rated their shock in stages of none, mild, medium, and severe. Individual StO_2 values were compared with each other.[78] StO_2 values were similar among groups, except that those in the severe shock state had significantly lower StO_2 values. However, most studies studying StO_2 values have demonstrated somewhat ambiguous results.[75,77] It seems that when a patient's StO_2 is consistently low for a period of time the presence of organ failure is also highly likely. Therefore, the use of NIRS in burn resuscitation cannot be recommended because of its overall unreliability and inconsistency of result.[79]

Gastric Tonometry

Gastric tonometry uses a silastic tube with saline pouch, placed into a patient's stomach, which then gathers samples from the gastric wall. These sample are then analyzed to determine a patient's CO_2 levels and ultimately perfusion. The CO_2 values change in response to hemodynamic challenges that alter blood flow in the gastrointestinal tract, providing a reasonable estimation of overall splanchnic perfusion.

Gastric tonometry has proven its effectiveness in the setting of trauma, sepsis, cardiac surgery, and critical care patients.[80,81] Conversely, studies have demonstrated no significant differences in data and patient outcomes with the use of gastric tonometry versus other previously mentioned methods for end point resuscitation.[82,83] This is most likely because when obtaining gastric tonometry measurements, the results are determined via a mathematical equation that measures a different CO_2 value (gastric) versus the direct measure of CO_2 in the bloodstream.[84] Thus, with this lack of reliability, it is difficult to promote the use of gastric tonometry as the sole tool in the identification of resuscitation end points.

Sublingual Capnometry

Sublingual capnometry is an alternative methodology of gastric tonometry developed with the purpose of using different locations than gastric tonometry to assess hypoperfusion in shock patients. This technique focuses uses the sublingual mucosa to gather Pco_2 values that are then translated into tissue perfusion levels in patients with hemorrhage and sepsis.[85,86] In trauma patients this tool seems to be capable of determining different levels of acute blood loss.[87] One study even demonstrated that sublingual tonometry was potentially capable of predicting survival in critically ill patients. However, these results were similar to those noted in previously mentioned studies using lactate and BD.[88] The paucity of data using sublingual capnometry makes it an experimental tool when guiding resuscitation efforts.[89]

SUMMARY

End points of resuscitation have been the subject of numerous strategies with conflicting results.[5–8,21] Many authors believe that urine output and traditional vital signs (heart rate and MAP) are too insensitive to ensure appropriate fluid replacement in burn injuries.[12,21] In children, trends in heart rate, blood pressure, and capillary refill toward normal are more reasonable therapeutic end points. In adults, arterial blood pressure is relatively insensitive to the adequacy of fluid replacement; pulse rate is more helpful. In older patients, pulse rate becomes less reliable. Urine output can be taken to reflect organ perfusion; however, urine must be nonglycosuric to be accurate.[17] Although urine output does not precisely mirror renal blood flow, it remains the most readily accessible and easily monitored index of resuscitation.[16,17] The definition of better end points of resuscitation to avoid excessive fluid administration is a priority for future study.[21] Multicenter studies to evaluate and establish these end points are paramount.[5,21]

ACKNOWLEDGMENTS

The authors wish to acknowledge the valuable contributions of Mr. Alexander Nolan regarding the content and presentation of this article.

REFERENCES

1. Gross SD. A system of surgery: pathological, diagnostic, therapeutic and operative. 4th edition. Philadelphia: H. C. Lea; 1866.
2. Blalock A. Shock: further studies with particular reference to the effects of hemorrhage. 1934. Arch Surg 2010;145(4):393–4.
3. Antonelli M, Levy M, Andrews PJ, et al. Hemodynamic monitoring in shock and implications for management. International Consensus Conference, Paris, France, April 2006. Intensive Care Med 2007;33(4):575–90.
4. American College of Surgeons, Committee on Trauma, ATLS. Advanced trauma life support for doctors. 8th edition. Chicago: American College of Surgeons; 2008. p. 366.
5. Ahrns KS. Trends in burn resuscitation: shifting the focus from fluids to adequate endpoint monitoring, edema control, and adjuvant therapies. Crit Care Nurs Clin North Am 2004;16:75–98.

6. Ipaktchi K, Arbabi S. Advances in burn critical care. Crit Care Med 2006;34: S239–44.

7. Barton RG, Saffle JR, Morris SE, et al. Resuscitation of thermally injured patients with oxygen transport criteria as goals of therapy. J Burn Care Rehabil 1997;18: 1–9.

8. Berger MM, Bernath MA, Chioléro RL. Resuscitation, anaesthesia and analgesia of the burned patient. Curr Opin Anaesthesiol 2001;14:431–5.

9. Demling RH. The burn edema process: current concepts. J Burn Care Rehabil 2005;26:207–27.

10. Rose JK, Herndon DN. Advances in the treatment of burn patients. Burns 1997; 23(Suppl 1):S19–26.

11. Warden GD. Burn shock resuscitation. World J Surg 1992;16:16–23.

12. Ahrns KS, Harkins DR. Initial resuscitation after burn injury: therapies, strategies, and controversies. AACN Clin Issues 1999;10:46–60.

13. Csontos C, Foldi V, Fischer T, et al. Factors affecting fluid requirement on the first day after severe burn trauma. ANZ J Surg 2007;77:745–8.

14. Willis MS, Carlson DL, DiMaio JM, et al. Macrophage migration inhibitory factor mediates late cardiac dysfunction after burn injury. Am J Physiol Heart Circ Physiol 2005;288:H795–804.

15. Maass DL, White J, Horton J. IL-1 beta and IL-6 act synergistically with TNF-alpha to alter cardiac contractile function after burn trauma. Shock 2002;18:360–6.

16. Pruitt BA. Advances in fluid therapy and the early care of the burn patient. World J Surg 1978;2:139–50.

17. Oliver RI, Spain D, Stadelmann W. Burns, resuscitation and early management. Available at: http://www.emedicine.com/plastic/topic159.htm. Accessed February 4, 2008.

18. Evans EI, Purnell OJ, Robinett PW, et al. Fluid and electrolyte requirements in severe burns. Ann Surg 1952;135:804–15.

19. Judkins K. Current consensus and controversies in major burns management. Trauma 2000;2:239–51.

20. Pham TN, Cancio LC, Gibran NS. American Burn Association practice guidelines burn shock resuscitation. J Burn Care Res 2008;29:257–66.

21. Latenser BA. Critical care of the burn patient: the first 48 hours. Crit Care Med 2009;37(10):2819–26.

22. Rivers E, Nguyen B, Havstad S, et al. Early goal-directed therapy in the treatment of severe sepsis and septic shock. N Engl J Med 2001;345(19):1368–77.

23. Donnino MW, Jørgensen NB, Jacobsen G, et al. Cryptic septic shock: a subanalysis of early, goal-directed therapy. Chest 2003;124 (90S–90b).

24. Dellinger RP, Levy MM, Rhodes A, et al. Surviving sepsis campaign: international guidelines for management of severe sepsis and septic shock, 2012. Intensive Care Med 2013;39(2):165–228.

25. Schiller WR, Bay RC. Hemodynamic and oxygen transport monitoring in management of burns. New Horiz 1996;4:475–81.

26. Schiller WR, Bay RC, Garren RL, et al. Hyperdynamic resuscitation improves survival in patients with life-threatening burns. J Burn Care Rehabil 1997;18:10–6.

27. Shoemaker WC, Appel PI, Kram HB, et al. Prospective trial of supranormal values of survivors as therapeutic goals in high risk surgical patients. Chest 1998;94: 1176–86.

28. Gattinoni L, Brazzi L, Pelosi P, et al. A trial of goal-oriented hemodynamic therapy in critically illpatients. SvO2 Collaborative Group. N Engl J Med 1995;333(16): 1025–32.

29. Durham RM, Neunaber K, Mazuski JE, et al. The use of oxygen consumption and delivery as endpoints for resuscitation in critically ill patients. J Trauma 1996; 41(1):32–9 [discussion: 39–40].
30. Velmahos GC, Demetriades D, Shoemaker WC, et al. Endpoints of resuscitation of critically injured patients: normal or supranormal? A prospective randomized trial. Ann Surg 2000;232(3):409–18.
31. Venkatesh B, Meacher R, Muller MJ, et al. Monitoring tissue oxygenation during resuscitation of major burns. J Trauma 2001;50:485–94.
32. Mansfield MD, Kinsella J. Use of invasive cardiovascular monitoring in patients with burns greater than 30 per cent body surface area: a survey of 251 centers. Burns 1996;22:549–51.
33. Reinhart K, Kuhn HJ, Hartog C, et al. Continuous central venous and pulmonary artery oxygen saturation monitoring in the critically ill. Intensive Care Med 2004; 30(8):1572–8.
34. Kopterides P, Bonovas S, Mavrou I, et al. Venous oxygen saturation and lactate gradient from superior vena cava to pulmonary artery in patients with septic shock. Shock 2009;31(6):561–7.
35. De Backer D, Ospina-Tascon G, Salgado D, et al. Monitoring the microcirculation in the critically ill patient: current methods and future approaches. Intensive Care Med 2010;36(11):1813–25.
36. Trzeciak S, Rivers EP. Clinical manifestations of disordered microcirculatory perfusion in severe sepsis. Crit Care 2005;9(Suppl 4):S20–6.
37. Rivers EP, Ander DS, Powell D. Central venous oxygen saturation monitoring in the critically ill patient. Curr Opin Crit Care 2001;7(3):204–11.
38. Ander DS, Jaggi M, Rivers E, et al. Undetected cardiogenic shock in patients with congestive heart failure presenting to the emergency department. Am J Cardiol 1998;82(7):888–91.
39. Scalea TM, Holman M, Fuortes M, et al. Central venous blood oxygen saturation: an early, accurate measurement of volume during hemorrhage. J Trauma 1988; 28(6):725–32.
40. Pinsky MR. Hemodynamic evaluation and monitoring in the ICU. Chest 2007; 132(6):2020–9.
41. Marik PE, Cavallazzi R, Vasu T, et al. Dynamic changes in arterial waveform derived variables and fluid responsiveness in mechanically ventilated patients: a systematic review of the literature. Crit Care Med 2009;37(9):2642–7.
42. Michard F, Boussat S, Chemla D, et al. Relation between respiratory changes in arterial pulse pressure and fluid responsiveness in septic patients with acute circulatory failure. Am J Respir Crit Care Med 2000;162(1):134–8.
43. Zhang Z, Lu B, Sheng X, et al. Accuracy of stroke volume variation in predicting fluid responsiveness: a systematic review and meta-analysis. J Anesth 2011; 25(6):904–16.
44. Zimmermann A, Kufner C, Hofbauer S, et al. The accuracy of the Vigileo/FloTrac continuous cardiac output monitor. J Cardiothorac Vasc Anesth 2008;22(3): 388–93.
45. Tsai YF, Liu FC, Yu HP. FloTrac/Vigileo system monitoring in acute-care surgery: current and future trends. Expert Rev Med Devices 2013;10(6):717–28.
46. Sundar S, Panzica P. LiDCO systems. Int Anesthesiol Clin 2010;48(1):87–100.
47. Oren-Grinberg A. The PiCCO monitor. Int Anesthesiol Clin 2010;48(1):57–85.
48. Benes J, Chytra I, Altmann P, et al. Intraoperative fluid optimization using stroke volume variation in high risk surgical patients: results of prospective randomized study. Crit Care 2010;14(3):R118.

49. Cecconi M, Fasano N, Langiano N, et al. Goal-directed haemodynamic therapy during elective total hip arthroplasty under regional anaesthesia. Crit Care 2011;15(3):R132.

50. Pearse R, Dawson D, Fawcett J, et al. Early goal-directed therapy after major surgery reduces complications and duration of hospital stay. A randomized, controlled trial [ISRCTN38797445]. Crit Care 2005;9(6):R687–93.

51. Manasia AR, Nagaraj HM, Kodali RB, et al. Feasibility and potential clinical utility of goal-directed transthoracic echocardiography performed by noncardiologist intensivists using a small hand-carried device (SonoHeart) in critically ill patients. J Cardiothorac Vasc Anesth 2005;19(2):155–9.

52. Huntsman LL, Stewart DK, Barnes SR, et al. Noninvasive Doppler determination of cardiac output in man. Clinical validation. Circulation 1983;67(3):593–602.

53. Monnet X, Rienzo M, Osman D, et al. Esophageal Doppler monitoring predicts fluid responsiveness in critically ill ventilated patients. Intensive Care Med 2005;31(9):1195–201.

54. Feissel M, Michard F, Faller JP, et al. The respiratory variation in inferior vena cava diameter as a guide to fluid therapy. Intensive Care Med 2004;30(9):1834–7.

55. Ferrada P, Anand RJ, Whelan J, et al. Qualitative assessment of the inferior vena cava: useful tool for the evaluation of fluid status in critically ill patients. Am Surg 2012;78(4):468–70.

56. Barbier C, Loubieres Y, Schmit C, et al. Respiratory changes in inferior vena cava diameter are helpful in predicting fluid responsiveness in ventilated septic patients. Intensive Care Med 2004;30(9):1740–6.

57. Vieillard-Baron A, Mayo PH, Vignon P, et al. Expert round table on echocardiography in ICU. International consensus statement on training standards for advanced critical care echocardiography. Intensive Care Med 2014;40(5): 654–66.

58. Levy B. Lactate and shock state: the metabolic view. Curr Opin Crit Care 2006; 12(4):315–21.

59. Jones AE, Shapiro NI, Trzeciak S, et al. Lactate clearance vs central venous oxygen saturation as goals of early sepsis therapy: a randomized clinical trial. JAMA 2010;303(8):739–46.

60. McNelis J, Marini CP, Jurkiewicz A, et al. Prolonged lactate clearance is associated with increased mortality in the surgical intensive care unit. Am J Surg 2001; 182(5):481–5.

61. Jansen TC, van Bommel J, Schoonderbeek FJ, et al. Early lactate-guided therapy in intensive care unit patients: a multicenter, open-label, randomized controlled trial. Am J Respir Crit Care Med 2010;182(6):752–61.

62. Consoli A, Nurjhan N, Reilly JJ Jr, et al. Contribution of liver and skeletal muscle to alanine and lactate metabolism in humans. Am J Physiol 1990;259(5 Pt 1): E677–84.

63. Connor H, Woods HF, Ledingham JG, et al. A model of L(1)-lactate metabolism in normal man. Ann Nutr Metab 1982;26(4):254–63.

64. Rutherford EJ, Morris JA Jr, Reed GW, et al. Base deficit stratifies mortality and determines therapy. J Trauma 1992;33(3):417–23.

65. Mutschler M, Nienaber U, Brockamp T, et al. Renaissance of base deficit for the initial assessment of trauma patients: a base deficit-based classification for hypovolemic shock developed on data from 16,305 patients derived from the Trauma Register DGU(R). Crit Care 2013;17(2):R42.

66. Davis JW, Parks SN, Kaups KL, et al. Admission base deficit predicts transfusion requirements and risk of complications. J Trauma 1996;41(5):769–74.

67. Eberhard LW, Morabito DJ, Matthay MA, et al. Initial severity of metabolic acidosis predicts the development of acute lung injury in severely traumatized patients. Crit Care Med 2000;28(1):125–31.
68. Dunham CM, Watson LA, Cooper C. Base deficit level indicating major injury is increased with ethanol. J Emerg Med 2000;18(2):165–71.
69. Brill SA, Stewart TR, Brundage SI, et al. Base deficit does not predict mortality when secondary to hyperchloremic acidosis. Shock 2002;17(6):459–62.
70. Chawla LS, Nader A, Nelson T, et al. Utilization of base deficit and reliability of base deficit as a surrogate for serum lactate in the peri-operative setting. BMC Anesthesiol 2010;10:16.
71. Chawla LS, Jagasia D, Abell LM, et al. Anion gap, anion gap corrected for albumin, and base deficit fail to accurately diagnose clinically significant hyperlactatemia in critically ill patients. J Intensive Care Med 2008;23(2):122–7.
72. Jeng JC, Jablonski K, Bridgeman A, et al. Serum lactate, not base deficit, rapidly predicts survival after major burns. Burns 2002;28:161–6.
73. Pal JD, Victorino GP, Twomey P, et al. Admission serum lactate levels do not predict mortality in the acutely injured patient. J Trauma 2006;60:583–9.
74. Vincent JL. End-points of resuscitation: arterial blood pressure, oxygen delivery, blood lactate, or …? Intensive Care Med 1996;22:3–5.
75. Santora RJ, Moore FA. Monitoring trauma and intensive care unit resuscitation with tissue hemoglobin oxygen saturation. Crit Care 2009;13(Suppl 5):S10.
76. Creteur J, Carollo T, Soldati G, et al. The prognostic value of muscle StO$_2$ in septic patients. Intensive Care Med 2007;33(9):1549–56.
77. Gomez H, Torres A, Polanco P, et al. Use of non-invasive NIRS during a vascular occlusion test to assess dynamic tissue O(2) saturation response. Intensive Care Med 2008;34(9):1600–7.
78. Skarda DE, Mulier KE, Myers DE, et al. Dynamic near-infrared spectroscopy measurements in patients with severe sepsis. Shock 2007;27(4):348–53.
79. Crookes BA, Cohn SM, Bloch S, et al. Can near-infrared spectroscopy identify the severity of shock in trauma patients? J Trauma 2005;58(4):806–13 [discussion: 813–6].
80. Kirton OC, Windsor J, Wedderburn R, et al. Failure of splanchnic resuscitation in the acutely injured trauma patient correlates with multiple organ system failure and length of stay in the ICU. Chest 1998;113(4):1064–9.
81. Marik PE. Gastric intramucosal pH. A better predictor of multiorgan dysfunction syndrome and death than oxygen-derived variables in patients with sepsis. Chest 1993;104(1):225–9.
82. Mythen MG, Webb AR. Perioperative plasma volume expansion reduces the incidence of gut mucosal hypoperfusion during cardiac surgery. Arch Surg 1995; 130(4):423–9.
83. Miami Trauma Clinical Trials Group. Splanchnic hypoperfusion-directed therapies in trauma: a prospective, randomized trial. Am Surg 2005;71(3):252–60.
84. Hameed SM, Cohn SM. Gastric tonometry: the role of mucosal pH measurement in the management of trauma. Chest 2003;123(5 Suppl):475S–81S.
85. Creteur J. Gastric and sublingual capnometry. Curr Opin Crit Care 2006;12(3): 272–7.
86. Marik PE. Sublingual capnometry: a non-invasive measure of microcirculatory dysfunction and tissue hypoxia. Physiol Meas 2006;27(7):R37–47.
87. Creteur J, De Backer D, Sakr Y, et al. Sublingual capnometry tracks microcirculatory changes in septic patients. Intensive Care Med 2006;32(4):516–23.

88. Baron BJ, Sinert R, Zehtabchi S, et al. Diagnostic utility of sublingual PCO_2 for detecting hemorrhage in penetrating trauma patients. J Trauma 2004;57(1): 69–74.
89. Baron BJ, Dutton RP, Zehtabchi S, et al. Sublingual capnometry for rapid determination of the severity of hemorrhagic shock. J Trauma 2007;62(1):120–4.

Vitamin C in Burn Resuscitation

Julie A. Rizzo, MD[a,b],*, Matthew P. Rowan, PhD[a], Ian R. Driscoll, MD[a,b],
Kevin K. Chung, MD[a,b], Bruce C. Friedman, MD[c]

KEYWORDS

- Reactive oxygen species • Free radical • Ascorbic acid • Vitamin C • Burn

KEY POINTS

- Damage from reactive oxygen species significantly contributes to the increased resuscitative requirements after burn injury.
- Vitamin C is an inexpensive, readily available antioxidant.
- Preclinical and clinical studies demonstrate vitamin C can be an effective adjunct in burn resuscitation by decreasing overall fluid requirements and edema.
- Vitamin C appears to be well tolerated, but further investigation is needed to identify unanticipated effects from high-dose administration to burn patients.

INTRODUCTION

Proper fluid management in the immediate phase after significant burn injury is important for optimizing outcomes. The goal of burn resuscitation is to ensure adequate end-organ perfusion at the lowest physiologic cost. The pathophysiology of the massive fluid shifts that occur after burn injury and the underlying microvascular changes have been studied previously in an attempt to identify targets to reduce overall fluid requirements.[1–3] Increased capillary permeability results in the escape of fluid and protein from the intravascular into the interstitial space and is greatest in the first 8 hours after burn injury.[4] Compared with other forms of traumatic injury, the increased

The authors have nothing to disclose.
DOD Disclaimer: The opinions or assertions contained herein are the private views of the authors and are not to be construed as official or as reflecting the views of the Department of the Army or the Department of Defense. The views expressed herein are those of the authors and do not reflect the official policy or position of Brooke Army Medical Center, the US Army Medical Department, the US Army Office of the Surgeon General, the Department of the Army, and Department of Defense, or the US Government.
[a] United States Army Institute of Surgical Research, 3698 Chambers Pass, JBSA Fort Sam Houston, TX 78234, USA; [b] Department of Surgery, Uniformed Services University of the Health Sciences, 4301 Jones Bridge Road, Bethesda, MD 20814, USA; [c] JM Still Burn Center at Doctor's Hospital, 3651 Wheeler Road, Augusta, GA 30909, USA
* Corresponding author.
E-mail address: Julie.a.rizzo.mil@mail.mil

resuscitative requirements after burn injury are largely due to intravascular volume losses from capillary leakage. Excess fluid can accumulate in any tissue bed, resulting in resuscitation-related morbidity. These morbidities include pulmonary edema, compartment syndromes (muscle compartments, abdomen, and the orbits), and even cerebral edema.

Various inflammatory mediators have been shown to contribute to increased vascular permeability after burn injury, but mediator-targeted therapies have largely been unable to significantly mitigate capillary leak and thus decrease the resuscitation volumes needed. Reactive oxygen species (ROS) have also been reported to make a significant contribution to the increased vascular permeability, and antioxidant therapy has been investigated as a potential therapy to decrease ROS-induced damage. However, the pathophysiology of ROS-mediated damage and its effect on vascular permeability is complex and requires further investigation.

PATHOPHYSIOLOGY: INCREASED CAPILLARY PERMEABILITY

Increased capillary permeability after burn injury is due to several mechanisms. Immediately after a burn, mast cells release histamine that increases the activity of xanthine oxidase, which is one of many pathways that contribute to the increased production of ROS observed after burn injury.[2] ROS are formed endogenously during the metabolism of oxygen and can be produced through a variety of different enzymatic pathways, including NADPH oxidase, xanthine oxidase, and endothelial nitric oxide synthase, and in the electron transport chain.[5] ROS have vital physiologic roles in cell signaling, immune defense, and vascular tone, among others, but can also damage proteins, lipids, and nucleic acids at higher concentrations and have been implicated in many disease processes, such as cancer, insulin resistance, and atherosclerosis.[6] ROS-induced endothelial damage to lipids and proteins of cell membranes has been shown to contribute to the increased capillary leakage associated with burn injury.[7–10]

ANTIOXIDANT THERAPY

Therapies targeted at blocking the action of xanthine oxidase to reduce the formation of ROS have shown improved survival in preclinical burn models only when inhibitors are administered before burn injury,[11] which suggests that redundant formation pathways and enzyme activity create a complex barrier for effective targeting of ROS production. Therefore, a better strategy for preventing or minimizing increases in capillary permeability following burn injury might be to attenuate ROS-induced damage by removing ROS from circulation with a scavenger.[2,12] Therapies scavenging ROS as an adjunct in burn resuscitation could minimize capillary leak, and in turn, reduce the resuscitative requirements of large burns and minimize edema.

Because excess ROS is damaging to lipids, proteins, and nucleic acids, multiple endogenous systems exist to reduce ROS levels and include enzymes such as superoxide dismutase, catalase, peroxiredoxin, and thioredoxins.[12] For example, superoxide dismutase is part of an antioxidant system shown to decrease lipid peroxidation, a process that propagates chain reaction production of ROS.[13] However, the excessive ROS levels produced following a burn injury overwhelm endogenous systems, and exogenous ROS scavengers are needed to reduce ROS levels. Antioxidants are a class of effective ROS scavengers that act as reducing agents and become oxidized to neutralize ROS. Examples of nonenzymatic antioxidants include vitamins (such as C and E), minerals (such as selenium), and glutathione.[14] Several antioxidant therapies have been evaluated for their efficacy at reducing the capillary permeability after burn injury. Early administration of the histamine-blocker cimetidine reduced resuscitation requirements in thermally injured animals,[15] and further study suggested antioxidant, ROS-scavenging activity may be responsible for the beneficial effects of cimetidine.[2]

VITAMIN C

Ascorbic acid, or vitamin C, is a naturally occurring, essential nutrient that acts as an effective antioxidant and ROS scavenger. Vitamin C is highly water soluble and therefore cannot directly scavenge ROS within the cell membrane, but rather vitamin C removes ROS present in the extracellular space, thus regenerating vitamin E as a potent cell membrane ROS scavenger.[14] Vitamin C also protects circulating cells (erythrocytes and leukocytes) from ROS damage.[16] The high water solubility of vitamin C allows excess to be excreted by the kidney, preventing toxic accumulation.[17] The antioxidant effects of vitamin C have been studied as an adjunct in treating sepsis and ischemia/reperfusion injuries, where it was shown to improve tissue oxygenation and mitigate subsequent organ dysfunction.[18,19]

VITAMIN C: PRECLINICAL BURN STUDIES

Early reports of using vitamin C in burn injury demonstrated benefit in treating ocular alkali burns in a rabbit model[20] and in attenuating burn wound tissue necrosis when administered in the intraperitoneal space.[21] Preclinical studies have since evaluated the utility of vitamin C as an adjunct to burn resuscitation with the objective of decreasing total intravenous fluid requirement after a large burn (**Table 1**). In a guinea pig model of large burn (70% total body surface area [TBSA] burn), administration of high-dose vitamin C (14.2 mg/kg/h) effectively reduced the total fluid requirement while not compromising the hemodynamic parameters of the animals.[16,22–25] In fact, the cardiac output increased in direct proportion to a hematocrit decrease when vitamin C was administered within 6 hours of burn injury and for a duration of at least 6 hours.[4] Burn wound edema was significantly decreased after vitamin C administration,[16,22–25] and further studies demonstrated that the decrease in the strongly negative interstitial fluid hydrostatic pressure, lymph flow, and loss of protein from the interstitial space were, at least in part, responsible for the observed decrease in edema.[26,27] These findings have been reproduced in a large animal burn model where sheep (40% TBSA burn) given high-dose vitamin C (15 mg/kg/h) needed 30% less fluid at 6 hours and approximately 50% less fluid at 48 hours while maintaining adequate hemodynamics.[28] Furthermore, animals demonstrated decreased levels of plasma thiobarbituric acid reactive substances, an index of reduced lipid peroxidation.[28] Although most of the preclinical studies of vitamin C in burn models have been from one group, they nonetheless provide the framework for clinical investigations.

VITAMIN C: CLINICAL BURN STUDIES

To date, only 2 clinical studies have examined the utility of vitamin C as an adjunct in burn resuscitation. The first, published in 2000[29] by the same group that performed most of the preclinical studies, prospectively randomized 37 patients with greater than 30% TBSA thermal injury to isotonic and colloid fluid resuscitation with or without high-dose vitamin C (66 mg/kg/h). The Parkland formula was used to calculate expected fluid requirements, adding 5% albumin during the second and third 24 hours after injury. The vitamin C group required 45% less fluid at the 24-hour mark and demonstrated decreased lipid peroxidation, as evidenced by decreased serum

Table 1
Summary of preclinical studies of vitamin C in burn models

Lead Author, Year	Animal	Resuscitation (mL/kg/TBSA)	Vitamin C Dose (mg/kg/h)	Vitamin C Timing (h Postburn)	Findings in Vitamin C Patients
Matsuda et al,[23] 1991	Guinea pig	1–4	7–28.3	0.5–24	↑CO, ↓Hct, ↓skin H_2O content
Matsuda et al,[22] 1992	Guinea pig	1–4	7	0.5–24	↑CO, ↓Hct, ↓skin H_2O content
Matsuda et al,[26] 1992	Dog	Maintenance	14.2	0.25–6	↓Protein loss, ↓lymph flow
Tanaka et al,[4] 1992	Guinea pig	1–4	14.2	2–4, 2–8, 2–24	↑CO, ↓Hct
Tanaka et al,[24] 1995	Guinea pig	1–4	14.2	2–24	↑CO, ↓Hct
Matsuda et al,[16] 1995	Guinea pig	1–4	14.2	0.5–4, 0.5–8, 0.5–24	↑CO (peak at 8 h), ↓Hct (best at 8 h)
Tanaka et al,[25] 1997	Guinea pig	1–4	14.2	0.5–24	↑CO, ↓Hct, ↓burned skin H_2O content
Sakurai et al,[17] 1997	Guinea pig	1–4	14.2	6–24	↑CO, ↓Hct, ↓burned skin H_2O content
Tanaka et al,[27] 1999	Rat	?	33 (66 bolus)	(−)0.5–0.5	↓Pif, ↓total tissue H_2O content
Dubick et al,[28] 2005	Sheep	4	15	1–24	↓Net fluid, ↓plasma TBARS

Abbreviations: CO, cardiac output; Hct, hematocrit; Pif, interstitial fluid hydrostatic pressure; TBARS, thiobarbituric acid.

malondialdehyde levels compared with the non-vitamin C group. Respiratory function was also improved in the vitamin C patients with improved oxygenation and decreased duration of mechanical ventilation. However, this preliminary study did not show a significant difference in mortality.

The second clinical study[30] was a retrospective analysis of patients treated over a 3-year period (2007–2009) who were split into a control group, who were resuscitated according to the Parkland formula, and an experimental group, whose resuscitation strategy included the Parkland formula plus the volume required to achieve a vitamin C dose of 66 mg/kg/h, which for a 70-kg patient was an additional 168 mL/h. The 24-hour fluid requirements were 25% less in the vitamin C–treated subjects, and a diuresis was noted in this group as well, which decreased the net balance of fluid. Even though this study did not demonstrate improved respiratory function or improved mortality, which could be attributed to the small sample size, it did demonstrate that vitamin C could be used to decrease the overall resuscitation volume needed without an increased risk of renal failure or other infectious processes.

VITAMIN C: MECHANISMS OF ACTION IN BURN INJURY

In addition to ROS scavenging, regeneration of vitamin E, and attenuation of lipid per-oxidation, vitamin C functions through mechanisms specific to burn injury to decrease fluid requirements and wound edema. Because a reduced volume of isotonic fluid is required for burn patients treated with vitamin C, the dilutional hypoproteinemia causing decreased oncotic pressure and subsequent fluid shift into nonburned tissue is minimized,[31] evidenced in preclinical studies by a reduced water content in un-burned skin.[22] Wound edema is further decreased by vitamin C infusion through the inhibition of collagen denaturation and enhancement of hyaluronic acid removal, both of which have been shown to promote wound edema.[27,32,33] In addition, vitamin C affords protection to burned tissue capillary endothelium, which has been compromised by thermal injury, by scavenging ROS from the extracellular space.[4] Lower resuscitation volumes are often associated with a reduced incidence of intra-abdominal hypertension, which, in turn, has the potential to prevent abdominal compartment syndrome.[34,35]

VITAMIN C: SIDE EFFECTS

Vitamin C is highly hydrophilic and is readily excreted by the kidneys, thereby reducing potential toxicity that would be associated with elevated circulating concentrations. Literature evaluating the potential toxicity profile or side effects from high-dose vitamin C therapy is scarce, possibly because of the intravenous administration being so well tolerated. Because excess vitamin C is excreted by the kidneys, osmotic diuresis and worsening acute kidney injury have been identified as side effects in burn patients.[36] The intravenous formulation of vitamin C is hyperosmolar,[30] unless specific effort is made to create an isotonic, diluted solution.[29] Osmotic diuresis necessitates extra precautions be taken to ensure that acute kidney injury or hypovolemia does not occur as a result in resuscitated burn patients, so monitoring of serial hematocrit levels and evaluation for clinical signs of hypovolemia are vital.[30] Absorbed vitamin C is metab-olized to threose and oxalic acid, so oxalate nephropathy from a buildup of water-insoluble calcium oxalate has been demonstrated when vitamin C has been used as an alternative therapy for cancer and amyloidosis.[37,38] Oxalate nephropathy has also been observed in the postmortem examinations of a small number of burned pa-tients treated with high-dose (66 mg/kg/h) vitamin C as a rescue therapy during diffi-cult resuscitations.[39] Hyperoxaluria from high-dose vitamin C can worsen existing kidney injury or delay kidney recovery.[36] Renal toxicity should be carefully monitored in future studies, especially in patients with pre-existing kidney injury.

Another concern with vitamin C administration is the false elevation of point-of-care (POC) glucose measurements that has been reported.[40] In vitro studies have estab-lished that vitamin C interferes with electrochemical assays used to test POC glucose measurements[41] and that standard laboratory measurements have been necessary to determine accurate glucose levels for up to 24 hours after discontinuation of vitamin C infusion.

VITAMIN C: DOSING

The recommended adult daily intake of vitamin C is 75 mg for women and 90 mg for men. Because of high water solubility and low metabolism, daily oral doses of up to 10 g seem to be well tolerated. However, the optimal dosing of vitamin C in burn resus-citation has not been determined. Preclinical studies have examined doses of vitamin C ranging from 7 to 28.3 mg/kg/h and found efficacy in reducing resuscitation volume with a dose of 14.2 mg/kg/h.[23] The dose chosen for the 2 existing human studies was 66 mg/kg/h,[29,30] which is roughly 5-fold higher than that used in guinea pigs (14.2 mg/kg/h). It is unclear why 66 mg/kg/h was chosen for clinical studies, especially with respect to preclinical investigations that used substantially lower doses. The justification behind a higher dose for human studies seems to rely on the fact that larger mammals may need larger doses of vitamin C due to the more complex nature of ROS generating systems,[42] but controlled, dose-response studies have not yet been conducted to determine if lower doses would be equally effective at improving outcomes. Although a vitamin C dose of 66 mg/kg/h has been well tolerated in the existing human studies, further investigation is needed because there may be a dose-dependent increase in the incidence of renal toxicity, especially in the presence of existing kidney injury.[36] For a 70-kg patient, 66 mg/kg/h would be roughly 4.6 g/h, and over a 24-hour resuscitation period could approach a total dose of 110 g of vitamin C, potentially increasing the risk for adverse effects.

SUMMARY

Vitamin C holds potential as a powerful adjunct in burn resuscitation but a scarcity of definitive literature demonstrating therapeutic efficacy on clinical outcomes, combined with an incompletely understood side-effect profile, limits widespread implementation by burn centers. However, studies to date have shown that vitamin C may be safe and decreases fluid requirement in the acute phase after burn injury. Robust multicenter trials are needed to fully characterize the potential impact of vitamin C as an adjunct in burn resuscitation.

REFERENCES

1. Brouhard BH, Carvajal HF, Linares HA. Burn edema and protein leakage in the rat. I. Relationship to time of injury. Microvasc Res 1978;15(2):221–8.
2. Friedl HP, Till GO, Trentz O, et al. Roles of histamine, complement and xanthine oxidase in thermal injury of skin. Am J Pathol 1989;135(1):203–17.
3. Ward PA, Till GO. Pathophysiologic events related to thermal injury of skin. J Trauma 1990;30(12 Suppl):S75–9.
4. Tanaka H, Broaderick P, Shimazaki S, et al. How long do we need to give antioxidant therapy during resuscitation when its administration is delayed for two hours? J Burn Care Rehabil 1992;13(5):567–72.
5. Droge W. Free radicals in the physiological control of cell function. Physiol Rev 2002;82(1):47–95.
6. Alfadda AA, Sallam RM. Reactive oxygen species in health and disease. J Biomed Biotechnol 2012;2012:936486.
7. Cetinkale O, Belce A, Konukoglu D, et al. Evaluation of lipid peroxidation and total antioxidant status in plasma of rats following thermal injury. Burns 1997;23(2):114–6.
8. Nguyen TT, Cox CS, Traber DL, et al. Free radical activity and loss of plasma antioxidants, vitamin E, and sulfhydryl groups in patients with burns: the 1993 Moyer Award. J Burn Care Rehabil 1993;14(6):602–9.
9. Till GO, Hatherill JR, Tourtellotte WW, et al. Lipid peroxidation and acute lung injury after thermal trauma to skin. Evidence of a role for hydroxyl radical. Am J Pathol 1985;119(3):376–84.
10. Youn YK, Lalonde C, Demling R. Oxidants and the pathophysiology of burn and smoke inhalation injury. Free Radic Biol Med 1992;12(5):409–15.

11. Saez JC, Ward PH, Gunther B, et al. Superoxide radical involvement in the pathogenesis of burn shock. Circ Shock 1984;12(4):229–39.

12. Li X, Fang P, Mai J, et al. Targeting mitochondrial reactive oxygen species as novel therapy for inflammatory diseases and cancers. J Hematol Oncol 2013;6:19.

13. Thomson PD, Till GO, Woolliscroft JO, et al. Superoxide dismutase prevents lipid peroxidation in burned patients. Burns 1990;16(6):406–8.

14. Niki E. Interaction of ascorbate and alpha-tocopherol. Ann N Y Acad Sci 1987; 498:186–99.

15. Boykin JV Jr, Crute SL, Haynes BW Jr. Cimetidine therapy for burn shock: a quantitative assessment. J Trauma 1985;25(9):864–70.

16. Matsuda T, Tanaka H, Reyes HM, et al. Antioxidant therapy using high dose vitamin C: reduction of postburn resuscitation fluid volume requirements. World J Surg 1995;19(2):287–91.

17. Sakurai M, Tanaka H, Matsuda T, et al. Reduced resuscitation fluid volume for second-degree experimental burns with delayed initiation of vitamin C therapy (beginning 6 h after injury). J Surg Res 1997;73(1):24–7.

18. Biesalski HK, McGregor GP. Antioxidant therapy in critical care–is the microcirculation the primary target? Crit Care Med 2007;35(9 Suppl):S577–83.

19. May JM. How does ascorbic acid prevent endothelial dysfunction? Free Radic Biol Med 2000;28(9):1421–9.

20. Nirankari VS, Varma SD, Lakhanpal V, et al. Superoxide radical scavenging agents in treatment of alkali burns. An experimental study. Arch Ophthalmol 1981;99(5):886–7.

21. Hollinshead MB, Spillert CR, Lazaro EJ. The beneficial effects of ascorbic acid on murine burns. J Burn Care Rehabil 1985;6(1):50–4.

22. Matsuda T, Tanaka H, Shimazaki S, et al. High-dose vitamin C therapy for extensive deep dermal burns. Burns 1992;18(2):127–31.

23. Matsuda T, Tanaka H, Williams S, et al. Reduced fluid volume requirement for resuscitation of third-degree burns with high-dose vitamin C. J Burn Care Rehabil 1991;12(6):525–32.

24. Tanaka H, Hanumadass M, Matsuda H, et al. Hemodynamic effects of delayed initiation of antioxidant therapy (beginning two hours after burn) in extensive third-degree burns. J Burn Care Rehabil 1995;16(6):610–5.

25. Tanaka H, Matsuda H, Shimazaki S, et al. Reduced resuscitation fluid volume for second-degree burns with delayed initiation of ascorbic acid therapy. Arch Surg 1997;132(2):158–61.

26. Matsuda T, Tanaka H, Hanumadass M, et al. Effects of high-dose vitamin C administration on postburn microvascular fluid and protein flux. J Burn Care Rehabil 1992;13(5):560–6.

27. Tanaka H, Lund T, Wiig H, et al. High dose vitamin C counteracts the negative interstitial fluid hydrostatic pressure and early edema generation in thermally injured rats. Burns 1999;25(7):569–74.

28. Dubick MA, Williams C, Elgjo GI, et al. High-dose vitamin C infusion reduces fluid requirements in the resuscitation of burn-injured sheep. Shock 2005;24(2): 139–44.

29. Tanaka H, Matsuda T, Miyagantani Y, et al. Reduction of resuscitation fluid volumes in severely burned patients using ascorbic acid administration: a randomized, prospective study. Arch Surg 2000;135(3):326–31.

30. Kahn SA, Beers RJ, Lentz CW. Resuscitation after severe burn injury using high-dose ascorbic acid: a retrospective review. J Burn Care Res 2011;32(1):110–7.

31. Demling RH, Kramer G, Harms B. Role of thermal injury-induced hypoproteinemia on fluid flux and protein permeability in burned and nonburned tissue. Surgery 1984;95(2):136–44.
32. Murad S, Grove D, Lindberg KA, et al. Regulation of collagen synthesis by ascorbic acid. Proc Natl Acad Sci U S A 1981;78(5):2879–82.
33. Onarheim H, Brofeldt BT, Gunther RA. Markedly increased lymphatic removal of hyaluronan from skin after major thermal injury. Burns 1996;22(3):212–6.
34. Ivy ME, Atweh NA, Palmer J, et al. Intra-abdominal hypertension and abdominal compartment syndrome in burn patients. J Trauma 2000;49(3):387–91.
35. Kirkpatrick AW, Ball CG, Nickerson D, et al. Intraabdominal hypertension and the abdominal compartment syndrome in burn patients. World J Surg 2009;33(6): 1142–9.
36. Alkhunaizi AM, Chan L. Secondary oxalosis: a cause of delayed recovery of renal function in the setting of acute renal failure. J Am Soc Nephrol 1996;7(11):2320–6.
37. Lawton JM, Conway LT, Crosson JT, et al. Acute oxalate nephropathy after massive ascorbic acid administration. Arch Intern Med 1985;145(5):950–1.
38. Wong K, Thomson C, Bailey RR, et al. Acute oxalate nephropathy after a massive intravenous dose of vitamin C. Aust N Z J Med 1994;24(4):410–1.
39. Buehner M, Pamplin J, Studer L, et al. Oxalate nephropathy after continuous infusion of high-dose vitamin C as an adjunct to burn resuscitation. J Burn Care Res 2015. [Epub ahead of print].
40. Sartor Z, Kesey J, Dissanaike S. The effects of intravenous vitamin C on point-of-care glucose monitoring. J Burn Care Res 2015;36(1):50–6.
41. Moatti-Sirat D, Velho G, Reach G. Evaluating in vitro and in vivo the interference of ascorbate and acetaminophen on glucose detection by a needle-type glucose sensor. Biosens Bioelectron 1992;7(5):345–52.
42. Tolmasoff JM, Ono T, Cutler RG. Superoxide dismutase: correlation with life-span and specific metabolic rate in primate species. Proc Natl Acad Sci U S A 1980; 77(5):2777–81.

Pediatric Burn Resuscitation

Tina L. Palmieri, MD

KEYWORDS

- Pediatric • Burn • Resuscitation • Outcomes • Assessment

KEY POINTS

- Children have different airway anatomy than adults, resulting in a higher incidence of upper airway obstruction due to edema.
- Because children have a greater body surface area to volume ratio they have higher intravenous fluid requirements per percent burn and are prone to the development of hypothermia.
- Children are often unable to verbalize their needs, making pain management difficult.
- Initial burn resuscitation influences the long-term outcomes of children with burn injury.

INTRODUCTION

Burn injury is the third leading cause of unintentional injury and death in children less than 9 years of age. In the United States from 2001 to 2010, 1,501,737 children sustained burn injuries and 5842 died.[1,2] Annually, nearly 10,000 children have severe permanent disability from thermal injury.[3] Burn injury is treated in emergency departments, pediatrician offices, urgent care centers, family medicine clinics, and burn centers. The long-term outcome of a burned child is related to the initial assessment and treatment. Appropriate treatment reduces complications, scarring, and need for future reconstruction; inappropriate therapy can result in permanent disabilities or death. A working knowledge of initial burn assessment and treatment in children is, therefore, important.

The epidemiology of burn injury differs between children and adults. In the United States, scald burns are the most common cause of burn injury in children, followed by contact and flame burns.[4] Mortality for burned children is highest in the 0 to 2-year-old age group, who have incompletely developed immune and organ systems. Conversely, the 15 to 21-year-old group has the lowest mortality after burn injury,

Disclosure Statement: No financial disclosures.
Division of Burn Surgery, Department of Surgery, University of California Davis, Shriners Hospital for Children Northern California, 2425 Stockton Boulevard, Suite 718, Sacramento, CA 95817, USA
E-mail address: tlpalmieri@ucdavis.edu

Crit Care Clin 32 (2016) 547–559
http://dx.doi.org/10.1016/j.ccc.2016.06.004
0749-0704/16/$ – see front matter © 2016 Elsevier Inc. All rights reserved.

criticalcare.theclinics.com

with a LD (lethal dose) of 50 (burn size at which 50% of patients die) of greater than 90%.[5] Hence, the practitioner must carefully consider age when treating children.

The initial evaluation and treatment of burned children, although using the basic tenets of adult burn resuscitation, is markedly different in several areas, including airway management, fluid resuscitation, and pharmacologic therapies. Children are not "little adults" and have unique physiologic, physical, and psychosocial needs. Specialized knowledge, treatment modalities, and equipment are required to address those needs. The purpose of this article is to provide a foundation for initial assessment and management in burned children.

PATIENT EVALUATION OR OVERVIEW
Differences Between Children and Adults

The appropriate treatment of children with burn injury hinges on understanding how children differ from adults. These issues are discussed in terms of airway, breathing, circulation, neurologic issues, and skin.

Airway
There are multiple differences between pediatric and adult airways.[6] First, children have shorter tracheas and their tracheas have smaller diameter, putting children at greater risk for airway obstruction than adults. Second, the pharynx is anterior, with its narrowest portion at the cricothyroid membrane, making intubation more difficult. Children may also have large tonsils, making intubation difficult.

Breathing
Lung development in children occurs until the age of 8 years; the damage caused by smoke may impact lung development and lung function. Children also lack the pulmonary reserve present in older children and adults. Asthma is prevalent in children and may be both induced and exacerbated by the inhalation of smoke. Fortunately, children can compensate for hypoxia by increasing their respiratory rate and work of breathing; however, when they decompensate, it is often sudden and complete. In children cardiac arrest is more frequently associated with acute respiratory failure than in adults.[7]

Circulation
Perhaps the most important differences between children and adults are related to the body surface area and skin thickness. Children have a greater body surface area to mass ratio than adults, making them more susceptible to hypothermia and increasing fluid resuscitation requirements compared with an adult for any size burn. In addition, the body surface area is distributed differently in children than in adults. Children have larger heads (approaching 18% total body surface area [TBSA]) and smaller legs (approximately 14% TBSA). The Lund Browder Chart (**Table 1**) is often used in burn

Table 1 Lund Browder chart						
Age (y)	0	1	5	10	15	Adult
A	9.5	8.5	6.5	5.5	4.5	3.5
B	2.75	3.25	4	4.5	4.5	4.75
C	2.5	2.5	2.75	3	3.25	3.5

Body surface area for anterior portion of a child. A is head, B is thigh, C is calf. To obtain calculation for circumferential element, double the number shown.

size estimations because it accounts for body surface area distribution in multiple ages.[8] Hence, children require more intravenous (IV) fluid per kilogram for any size burn than their adult counterparts.

The circulatory system in infants and children also differs from that of adults. Infants have limited cardiac contractility and, as such, can only increase cardiac output by increasing their heart rate. Tachycardia after burn injury is common and frequently not related to hypovolemia or pain, although these must still be considered in every tachycardic infant.

Neurologic

One of the hallmarks of childhood is neural development. As children grow, they go through developmental stages. Infants depend on caregivers, toddlers explore their environment, children have concrete thinking with increasing physical coordination and strength, and adolescents develop complex thinking yet experience hormone surges that may alter behavior. As such, the communication strategy must be different with each developmental phase.

Assessing pain and neurologic status is challenging in children because many cannot verbalize pain or anxiety. A variety of age-specific pain and anxiety scales exist and are used to guide care.[9,10] In general, a child should be upset and crying after burn injury. A moribund or minimally responsive child is likely to be in shock and requires immediate attention. Children who can verbalize should be encouraged to do so, and adolescents should be informed and involved in their own care.

Child abuse should always be considered in a child with burn injury, particularly in stoic children with a burn injury pattern that does not match the story given by the parent or in cases when delays in seeking treatment occur (**Box 1**).

Skin

Children's skin differs from that of adults. Because children have thinner skin, they will sustain a deeper burn at any given temperature. In addition, children have thinner skin with fewer appendages, which increases the likelihood of a third-degree burn injury.

Box 1
Child abuse risk factors

Pattern of injury is not compatible with the history given.

Account of injury cause changes over time.

A young sibling is blamed for the burn.

The caregiver was absent at the time of injury.

The lines of demarcation between normal and burned skin are straight or smooth

The burn is in a "glove" or "stocking" distribution.

Long delay between burn injury and seeking of treatment.

The caregiver is more concerned about themselves than the child.

The child is unusually passive when subjected to painful procedures.

Multiple burns of different ages are present.

Other forms of injury are present or siblings have similar injuries.

Lack of cleanliness, malnutrition, poor dentition.

History of previous Child Protective Services reports.

Because of their susceptibility to hypothermia, wet dressings should be avoided in children with burn injury.

Infants and children also have incompletely developed immune systems and have not been exposed to many virulent infections. As such, they are susceptible to infection and sepsis. Prophylactic antibiotics select out for virulent organisms and should be avoided in children with burns.

Initial Evaluation

History

The initial evaluation of every child with a burn injury should include obtaining history of the circumstances surrounding the thermal injury. The child's medical and birth history may also provide insight into potential complications. The history should be solicited from both the child and the caregiver.

The history of injury and the burn injury pattern should be evaluated for consistency and compared with the developmental age of the child. Infants, because they lack mobility and strength, are unable to escape heat. Toddlers tend to explore their environments with their hands and mouths, yet have not developed the protective reflex to pull away after contacting a hot surface. Toddlers often sustain burns to the palm and fingers as they grab or touch items. Toilet training is a high-risk time for "dip" burns associated with child abuse. High-risk behavior increases in children as they test boundaries; thus, children tend to suffer flame burns as they play with matches or accelerants. Peer pressure may increase risk-taking and suicide burns in teenagers.

Physical examination

Ultimately, the severity of any burn injury depends on age, body surface involvement (TBSA), and burn depth. The rule of nines used frequently in adults to estimate burn size is of less value in the young child. The Lund and Browder Chart (see **Table 1**) details body surface area distribution and assists in calculating the percentage of body at different ages. The child's palm (including fingers) is 1% of their body surface area, which can be used to assist in burn size estimations.

Initial Resuscitation

Airway

Fundamental airway principles after thermal and inhalation injuries have been discussed in previous chapters and will not be repeated. One issue more prevalent in children than adults is airway obstruction due to edema. As previously mentioned, a child's airway is smaller; hence, less edema is needed to develop airway obstruction. Signs of airway obstruction include hoarseness, increased work of breathing, tachypnea, and the use of accessory muscles. Owing to the smaller diameter of the child's airway, infants, younger children with larger burns, and those with face burns are particularly at risk. Endotracheal intubation is indicated in infants and children with significant airway compromise from edema involving the glottis and upper airway. Children will develop significant edema due to resuscitation even in the absence of a face burn. Hence, children with burns greater than 40% should be monitored closely for airway compromise.

If intubation is required, it should be performed by a practitioner experienced in managing the difficult pediatric airway. Endotracheal tube size is chosen based on the diameter of the child's external nares or small finger or by using the equation [16 + age in years]/4. Because the narrowest point of the child's airway is at the cricoid, surgical cricothyrotomy is contraindicated. In the rare occasion when an infant is in extremis and cannot be intubated, a needle cricothyrotomy may be used temporarily until a definitive airway can be obtained. After intubation, placement of a nasogastric tube is advisable because infants and children often develop gastric distension from swallowing air when crying.

Breathing
Children may have significant pulmonary damage due to smoke inhalation with few physical or radiographic signs in the first 24 hours after the burn. All children with suspected inhalation injury should be evaluated frequently for adequate air exchange. Children differ from adults in the extent and rapidity of tachypnea, their compliant chest wall, and the use abdominal musculature for breathing when stressed. Early intubation for signs of hypoxia or hypercarbia may prevent complications. However, intubation is not without risks, especially in children. Tube malposition, aspiration, and pneumonia are only a few of the complications of endotracheal intubation. It is essential that the practitioner confirm endotracheal tube placement after intubation. Children with significant respiratory injury should be transferred to a burn center experienced in pediatric burn care.

Circulatory status
After the airway has been secured, the child's circulatory status should be established. Hypovolemic infants are mottled, lethargic, and have dry mucous membranes. IV fluid resuscitation should be initiated promptly in infants with a burn encompassing greater than 15% TBSA. Delays in initiation of fluid resuscitation may result in longer hospital length of stay, increased complications, acute renal failure, and increased mortality.[11] Tachycardia is not a reliable sign of volume status in a burned child because tachycardia is a normal finding in a child with a burn size greater than 15%.

IV cannulae should be inserted percutaneously in a peripheral vein or by cut-down into burned or unburned skin. Adjuncts such as ultrasound may be helpful in placing peripheral IV catheters. Large-bore peripheral access is preferred because smaller catheters are unable to provide adequate fluid administration. Central venous catheterization is safe for children with massive burns. Intraosseous infusion may be lifesaving in the severely burned infant, but is indicated only when IV line placement has been unsuccessful. Intraosseous lines should be replaced with a more permanent access at the first opportunity and should be monitored closely because extremity compartment syndrome has resulted from misplaced intraosseous lines.

Children have unique fluid needs after burn injury. Ringer's Lactate solution should be started in patients of all age groups. In infants, hypoglycemia may develop owing to limited glycogen stores; therefore, blood glucose levels should be monitored. Glucose-free resuscitation fluids combined with maintenance fluids (MFs) with 5% dextrose should be administered to infants and young children (see later description).

The principles behind fluid resuscitation are similar for children and adults. The volume of fluid required per percent burn is higher in children owing to their increased baseline body surface area. Hence, pediatric burn resuscitation uses the adult burn formula and adds normal MF with dextrose. The resuscitation calculation for children includes both the estimated fluid resuscitation (EFR) needs (4 mL × weight [kg] × TBSA burn) and MFs to account for the increased body surface area of children.

Starting IV fluid rate in the infant and child (<20 kg) is estimated by the following:

Hourly IV fluid requirement = EFR + MF

EFR = 4 mL × weight (kg) × TBSA burn, half in the first 8 hours

Therefore, 8 hour total fluid volume = [4 mL × weight (kg) × TBSA burn]/2

Starting fluid rate per hour for the first 8 hours (divide by 8): [8 hour total fluid volume]/8

Plus

MF (hourly rate):

For the first 10 kg of body weight: (4 mL × kg)/h

For second 10 kg of body weight: (2 mL × kg)/h

For each kilogram of body weight more than 20 kg: (1 mL × kg)/h

Total MF rate is the sum of the above.

Resuscitation formulas are estimates. IV fluid rates need to be adjusted based on urinary output. In children weighing less than 30 kg, the urinary output goal is 1 mL/kg/h. In children over 30 kg, a urinary output of .5 mL/kg/h is the goal. Urine volumes less than or greater than this requires adjustment in fluid resuscitation rates. Only partial thickness (blistered) and full-thickness burns should be used to calculate the TBSA burn for the purpose of resuscitation. Adjuncts to monitoring urine output include assessment of sensorium, blood pH, and the peripheral circulation. Delays, underestimation of fluid requirements, and overestimation of fluid requirements may result in increased mortality.

Wound assessment

Although wounds are a major component of burn treatment, airway, breathing, and circulation management take precedence. As in adults, initial management of the burn wound includes stopping the burning process, removing all clothing, examining the entire body surface to determine the extent of the burn injury, and covering the burned areas immediately after inspection. The child's body temperature should be closely monitored and the ambient temperature in the examination room warm to decrease the incidence of hypothermia. Warm IV fluids and warm blankets are useful adjuncts in this setting. Wet dressings should not be applied because they increase the incidence of hypothermia. Extremities and the head, if burned, should be elevated to decrease edema.

As in adults, determination of wound area is important in guiding resuscitation. Children have a different body surface area distribution than adults (see **Table 1**). In general, children have larger heads and smaller thighs than adults. As mentioned above, the child's palm and fingers are 1% of their body surface area. This can be used to estimate burn size. In estimating burn size, only areas of second and third degree (blisters or eschar) should be included in the fluid resuscitation calculation.

If the patient will be transferred to a burn facility within 24 hours, topical antimicrobial dressings are not indicated before transfer. Application of clean, dry dressings to maintain body temperature is appropriate. If transfer is delayed, wound care topical antimicrobials, such as silver sulfadiazine or bacitracin, can be applied. During transfer, measures to conserve body heat, including thermal blankets, are essential for the infant and young child.

The chest wall is more compliant in children than in adults. Hence, children may become rapidly exhausted by the edema and restrictive effects of a circumferential chest wall burn. Likewise, the patient may develop abdominal compartment syndrome, which restricts lung expansion. Bladder pressures should be monitored and escharotomy performed if pressure exceeds 30 mm Hg.

PHARMACOLOGIC TREATMENT OPTIONS
Airway

There are limited options to decrease airway edema after burn and inhalation injury. Administration of steroids has not been shown to decrease airway edema, improve oxygenation, or decrease mortality. Steroids could potentially increase the risk of pneumonia and are thus contraindicated in burn inhalation injury. In patients with carboxyhemoglobin toxicity, treatment with 100% oxygen decreases carboxyhemoglobin levels and is recommended. The use of hyperbaric oxygen for combined burn or inhalation injury is controversial, at best, and has no proven benefit.

Breathing

Several different pharmacologic options are available for the treatment of inhalation injury in children. These therapies include the use of aerosolized heparin, tocopherol, and β2-agonists.[12–14] Aerosolized heparin purportedly decreases cast formation; however, patient antithrombin III levels need to be monitored because heparin is ineffective in the absence of antithrombin III. The nebulized agent albuterol has been shown to improve oxygenation and decrease ventilation pressures in inhalation sheep models; however, a prospective trial is needed to prove efficacy. Nitric oxide has been shown to decrease pulmonary hypertension and improve oxygenation in critically ill patients but has not improved outcomes after burn injury.[15–17] Further randomized prospective trials are needed to validate these therapies.

Circulation

The primary focus of treatment of the hypovolemic shock accompanying burn injury is IV fluid administration using lactated Ringer's solution. The use of vasopressors after burn injury is discouraged because most vasopressors cause cutaneous vasoconstriction and could potentiate the depth of the burn injury. Children with heart failure during the first 36 hours of resuscitation may benefit from cardiac inotropes if they have adequate filling pressures. Beta blockade has been advocated in the postresuscitation phase to decrease metabolic rate, but caution should be exercised during the resuscitation phase because nonspecific beta blockade can result in cardiac failure, exacerbation of pulmonary injury, and gastrointestinal ischemia. Anabolic agents, such as growth hormone and oxandrolone, have been shown to improve lean body mass, improve strength, and decrease length of stay after burn injury. These agents should be instituted after beginning enteral nutrition.[18,19]

Neurologic

Pain management and sedation in children with acute burn injury can be quite challenging. Children (and caregivers) may have difficulty distinguishing between pain and anxiety. Child-specific pain and anxiety scales should be used to guide therapy. Codeine should be avoided in children because it is not properly metabolized in approximately 30% of children.[20,21]

IV narcotics, such as morphine, should be used for acute pain management. Sedative agents useful in children include short-acting benzodiazepines. In general, intermittent dosing of narcotics and sedatives after burn injury should be used to decrease the fluid creep that accompanies continuous infusions. Recent reports of the use of ketamine and dexmedetomidine are promising, but additional studies are needed to confirm their efficacy.

Wound

Discussion of wound care is limited to those specific for children (see other sections of this missive.) In general, the choice of topical antimicrobial treatment of second-degree and third-degree burns in children is similar to that in adults. However, special care must be taken with the use of silver products in the newborn and children because silver can cause kernicterus in these populations. In general, simple dressings that can be left in place for several days (some of the topical silver dressings) and that are easy to remove are advisable for superficial partial thickness burns in children. For children who cannot tolerate silver-based products, topical gels such as bacitracin may be advisable.

NONPHARMACOLOGIC TREATMENT OPTIONS

There are several nonpharmacologic treatments that are essential in the resuscitation of the burned child, including physical and occupational therapy and nutrition.

Nutrition

A major burn injury causes a hypermetabolic response in children, which markedly increases caloric requirements.[22] In children with burn size greater than 40%, it is advisable to insert a nasoenteral tube and initiate feedings within the first 12 hours of injury. The hypermetabolic response continues throughout hospitalization and can last greater than 6 months. Recommended caloric intake is shown in **Table 2**. Weekly resting energy expenditure should be performed to adjust enteral nutrition.

Physical and Occupational Therapy

Burned children preferentially lose lean muscle mass after injury. In addition, children are often at bed rest due to multiple surgical procedures. Hence, weakness, muscle atrophy, and bone demineralization are common after major burn injury. Early mobilization, splinting, and exercise programs are the cornerstones of therapy after burn injury. Exercise programs have been shown to improve endurance, improve lean muscle mass, and improve outcomes in severely burned children.

Child Life and Distraction Therapies

A useful adjunct in the treatment of pain in children with burn injury is the use of child life therapists to educate child and family, help children develop coping

Table 2
Nutritional recommendations for children with burn injury

Category	Age (y)	Maintenance (kilograms)	+% Burn Calories per Day
Infants	0–1	98–108	+15 × TBSA
Children	1–3	102	+ 25 × TBSA
	4–6	90	+ 40 × TBSA
	7–10	70	+ 40 × TBSA
Adolescents			
Male	11–14	55	+ 40 × TBSA
	15–18	45	+ 40 × TBSA
Female	11–14	47	+ 40 × TBSA
	15–18	40	+ 40 × TBSA

Adapted from Chan MM, Chan GM, Nutritional therapy for burns in children and adults. Nutrition 2009;25(3):261–9; with permission.

skills, and provide distraction therapy during painful procedures to decrease the psychological impact of the burn injury. Other forms of distraction during dressing changes, such as virtual reality and computer gaming, have demonstrated some efficacy in decreasing pain and anxiety during burn dressing changes in children.[23,24]

COMBINATION THERAPIES

The treatment of a burned child is a team effort, combining the skills of multiple different professionals ranging from intensivists, surgeons, and nurses to therapists, dieticians, child life specialists, social workers, and psychologists. Each child's treatment will involve both pharmacologic and nonpharmacological therapies tailored to the child's needs. This team approach using a combination of therapies is essential to optimizing the outcomes of the burned child.

SURGICAL TREATMENT OPTIONS

Resuscitation is key to the child's survival and outcome after burn injury. Several surgical options are available and/or necessary in the resuscitative period, including escharotomy and early excision.

Escharotomy

Escharotomy may be required in the burned child, as in the adult, to relieve compartment syndrome of the extremities, chest, or abdomen. Although the basic tenets of escharotomy is similar for children and adults, escharotomy in children should only be performed by experienced burn surgeons. Children have thinner skin, smaller limbs, and different body fat distribution than adults. The margin for error is extremely small, especially in infants. Hypothermia may be exacerbated during escharotomy. Escharotomy is rarely required before burn center transfer. In children receiving massive fluid resuscitation or with electrical burns, fasciotomy may be necessary due to the relatively small size of the child's muscle compartments in each extremity. Again, this procedure should only be performed by experienced pediatric burn specialists.

Abdominal compartment syndrome may occur in children receiving massive fluid resuscitation or overresuscitation (in excess of 6 mL/kg/TBSA burn in <24 hours). The hallmark of abdominal compartment syndrome in children is abdominal distension, elevated intraabdominal pressures (>30 mm Hg), oliguria or anuria, and decreased ventilator tidal volumes. Exploratory laparotomy with placement of a negative pressure device (if no abdominal wall burn) or silastic sheet (if extensive abdominal wall burn) will relieve the compartment syndrome. When edema resolves, the abdomen can be closed.

Early Excision

Early excision of major burn injury decreases hospital length of stay, decreases infection rates, improves mortality, improves cardiac function, and decreases overall blood transfusions in children.[25–27]

In general, third-degree burns should be excised and grafted within 3 to 5 days of admission, if resources and expertise exist to do so. Autografting is the optimal coverage; however, in massive burns either allograft or skin substitutes may be used to temporize the wound bed until autograft donor sites become available.

TREATMENT RESISTANCE OR COMPLICATIONS
Airway

Airway obstruction due to edema is the most serious immediate life-threatening problem after inhalation injury or burn. Children have the same risk factors for upper airway obstruction due to edema as adults (inhalation injury, face burns, massive burns over 40% TBSA, prolonged extrication). Smaller children are particularly prone to acute airway obstruction compared with older children or adults owing to the smaller diameter of their airway. For example, 1 mm of edema in an infant with a 4 mm airway will decrease the cross-sectional area of the trachea by 75% and increase resistance 16-fold. In an adult with an 8 mm airway, the cross-section area would only be reduced by 44% and resistance increased only 3-fold. Children develop edema throughout their bodies in response to burns over 40% TBSA, and can develop airway obstruction even after a scald burn with no facial involvement. The child's airway needs to be meticulously evaluated frequently after major burn injury.

Breathing

As previously mentioned, a child's lungs continue to develop until the age of 8 years, and children have a higher incidence of reactive airway disease than adults. Hence, children are at increased risk for the development of acute respiratory distress syndrome and pneumonia, particularly after inhalation injury.

Circulation

The most common circulatory issues in children with major burn injury are either over-resuscitation or under-resuscitation. Resuscitation formulas should be used to initiate therapy. However, the IV fluid resuscitation rate should be reevaluated on an hourly basis and IV rate adjusted accordingly. In general, if a child has a urine output of greater than 1 mL/kg/h, the IV fluid infusion rate should be decreased by 10%. Conversely, if the child has a urine output of less than 0.8 mL/kg/h, IV fluids should be increased by 10%. Cardiac output decreases during the first 24 to 36 hours after major burn injury. Hence, children with burns greater than 40% TBSA should have advanced monitoring, including central venous pressures. Children receiving IV fluid rates twice that predicted by the Parkland formula, with continued inadequate urine output, are likely to have either heart failure or other complications of over-resuscitation, including abdominal compartment syndrome or pleural effusion. Under-resuscitation in children is generally due to either incorrect estimation of burn size or delays in obtaining intravascular access. The short length of pediatric IV catheters can lead to extravasation as the patient develops edema after burn injury. Central lines in children can compromise circulation to extremities and require expertise to insert. Intraosseous lines can result in limb loss due to compartment syndrome from either a misplaced or dislodged catheter, or leakage of infused fluids around the needle insertion site.

Neurologic

Pain management during resuscitation in burned children is particularly challenging. Children will be combative during wound care and dressing changes. Providers respond by administering narcotics and benzodiazepines. However, once the stimulus stops, children can be oversedated because the half-life of the drug is longer than the painful dressing change. Frequent administration of short-acting narcotics via IV or the use of the neuroleptic sedative agent ketamine (administered by trained providers) may ameliorate this issue.

A second neurologic issue unique to children with major burn injury is resuscitation-related cerebral edema. Although the cause is unclear, the principle is similar to airway issues: a child has a smaller diameter head than an adult, so pressure increases with smaller amounts of intracranial edema. There is laboratory evidence that the blood brain barrier may be violated after major burn injury and lead to neurologic dysfunction.[28]

Wound Infection or Poorly Healing Wounds

Although children have an amazing capacity to heal wounds, their immature immune system makes them susceptible to a wide variety of wound infections. Fever to 38.5°C is common after burn injury, making the diagnosis of infection difficult. Children who have dressing changes once or twice a week and children with deep partial thickness burns, in particular, may develop toxic shock syndrome or virulent streptococcal reaction. If this occurs, the dressing should be immediately removed and antibiotics administered via IV. In the event there is no improvement, operative excision may be indicated.

EVALUATION OF OUTCOME AND LONG-TERM RECOMMENDATIONS

Overall, there has been a marked improvement in survival for burned children in the past 40 years. The burn size resulting in 50% mortality (otherwise termed the LD50) for children with burn injury is greater than 90% TBSA burn. Highest survival is in the 5 to 15-year-old group. Children less than 2 years of age have a markedly higher mortality, likely due to their organ immaturity, inability to extricate themselves from the fire environment, and delays in care due to unavailability or inability to obtain appropriate medical devices (ie, difficulty in inserting an endotracheal tube or IV catheter because the size needed for an infant is not available). Early, appropriate airway and IV fluid administration in burns greater than 40% have been associated with improved outcomes. Delay in resuscitation of 2 hours has an adverse effect on survival and infection rates in children with burn injury.[11]

Another factor that may contribute to mortality is provider experience with pediatric burn injury treatment. Burned children require specialized equipment, as well as personnel who are trained or experienced in using the equipment in children and in the medical management of children in different developmental stages. The survival of children with burn injury has been linked to provider experience in several studies.[5,29]

Examination of long-term functional outcomes in burned children is necessary. Age-specific quality of life growth charts have been developed for important measures including functional activities, psychological adjustment, and social reintegration after burn injury.[30] Early resuscitation and management of burned children incorporating the principle "do it right the first time" will decrease the number and extent of reconstructive procedures as the child grows.

SUMMARY

Appropriate initial resuscitation is essential in optimizing both survival and functional outcomes in burned children. As such, initial resuscitation of the burned child should not only use a systematic approach to the pulmonary, circulatory, neurologic, and cutaneous aspects of injury but also adapt care to the unique physiologic and psychological needs of the burned child. Children with major burn injury greater than 20% should be stabilized and transferred to centers experienced in pediatric burn care.

REFERENCES

1. Borse NN, Gilchrist J, Dellinger AM, et al. CDC Childhood Injury Report: Patterns of unintentional injuries among 0-19 year olds in the United States, 2000–2006. Atlanta (GA): Division of Unintentional Injury Prevention, National Center for Injury Prevention and Control Centers for Disease Control and Prevention. Available at: http://www.cdc.gov/SafeChild/ChildhoodInjuryReport/index.html. Accessed June 15, 2014.

2. National Center for Injury Prevention and Control, CDC WISQARS injury incidence calculator. Fatal and nonfatal burn injuries 2001-11. Data from NEISS All Injury Program operated by the Consumer Product Safety Commission for numbers of injuries. Available at: http://webappa.cdc.gov/sasweb/ncipc/nfirates2001.html. Accessed July 2, 2014.

3. Advanced burn life support manual. Chicago: American Burn Association; 2007.

4. Saeman MR, Hodgman EI, Burris A, et al. Epidemiology and outcomes of pediatric burns over 35 years at Parkland Hospital. Burns 2016;42:202–8.

5. Palmieri TL, Taylor S, Lawless M, et al. Burn center volume makes a difference for burned children. Pediatr Crit Care Med 2015;16(4):319–24.

6. Santillanes G, Gausche-Hill M. Pediatric airway management. Emerg Med Clin North Am 2008;26(4):961–75.

7. Atkins DL, Berger S, Duff JP, et al. Part 11: pediatric basic life support and cardiopulmonary resuscitation quality: 2015 American Heart Association guidelines update for cardiopulmonary resuscitation and emergency cardiovascular care. Circulation 2015;132(18 Suppl 2):S519–25.

8. Lund CC, Browder NC. The estimation of areas of burns. Surgery, Gynaecology, Obstetrics 1944;79:352–8.

9. Playfor S, Jenkins I, Boyles C, et al. Consensus guidelines on sedation and analgesia in critically ill children. Intensive Care Med 2006;32:1125–36.

10. Willis MH, Merkel SI, Voepel-Lewis T, et al. FLACC Behavioral Pain Assessment Scale: a comparison with the child's self-report. Pediatr Nurs 2003;29:195–8.

11. Barrow RE, Jeschke MG, Herndon DN. Early fluid resuscitation improves outcomes in severely burned children. Resuscitation 2000;45(2):91–6.

12. Enkhbaatar P, Cox R, Traber LD, et al. Aerosolized anticoagulants ameliorate acute lung injury in sheep after exposure to burn and smoke inhalation. Crit Care Med 2007;12:2805–10.

13. Morita N, Traber MG, Enkhbaatar P, et al. Aerosolized alpha-tocopherol ameliorates acute lung injury following combined burn and smoke inhalation injury in sheep. Shock 2006;25:277–82.

14. Palmieri TL. Use of beta-agonists in inhalation injury. J Burn Care Res 2009;30:156–9.

15. Musgrave MA, Fingland R, Gomez M, et al. The use of inhaled nitric oxide as adjuvant therapy in patients with burn injuries and respiratory failure. J Burn Care Rehabil 2000;21(6):551–7.

16. Sheridan RL, Zapol WM, Ritz RH, et al. Low-dose inhaled nitric oxide in acutely burned children with profound respiratory failure. Surgery 1999;126(5):856–62.

17. Sheridan RL, Hurford WE, Kacmarek RM, et al. Inhaled nitric oxide in burn patients with respiratory failure. J Trauma 1997;42(4):629–34.

18. Abdullahi A, Jeschke MG. Nutrition and anabolic pharmacotherapies in the care of burn patients. Nutr Clin Pract 2014;29(5):621–30.

19. Diaz EC, Herndon DN, Porter C, et al. Effects of pharmacological interventions on muscle protein synthesis and breakdown in recovery from burns. Burns 2015; 41(4):649–57.
20. Tremlett M, Anderson BJ, Wolf A. Pro-con debate: is codeine a drug that still has a useful role in pediatric practice? Paediatr Anaesth 2010;20(2):183–94.
21. Kelly PA. Pharmacogenomics: why standard codeine doses can have serious toxicities or no therapeutic effect. Oncol Nurs Forum 2013;40(4):322–4.
22. Jeschke MG, Chinkes DL, Finnerty CC, et al. Pathophysiologic response to severe burn injury. Ann Surg 2008;248(3):387–401.
23. Kipping B, Rodger S, Miller K, et al. Virtual reality for acute pain reduction in adolescents undergoing burn wound care: a prospective randomized controlled trial. Burns 2012;38(5):650–7.
24. Parry I, Carbullido C, Kawada J, et al. Keeping up with video game technology: objective analysis of Xbox Kinect™ and PlayStation 3 Move™ for use in burn rehabilitation. Burns 2014;40:852–9.
25. Wu XW, Herndon DN, Spies M, et al. Effects of delayed wound excision and grafting in severely burned children. Arch Surg 2002;137:1049–54.
26. Pietsch JB, Netscher DT, Nagaraj HS, et al. Early excision of major burns in children: effect on morbidity and mortality. J Pediatr Surg 1985;20(6):754–7.
27. Barrett JP, Herndon DN. Effects of burn wound excision on bacterial colonization and invasion. Plast Reconstr Surg 2003;111(2):744–50.
28. Flierl MA, Stahel PF, Touban BM, et al. Bench-to-bedside review: burn-induced cerebral inflammation–a neglected entity? Crit Care 2009;13(3):215.
29. Sheridan RL, Weber JM, Schnitzer JJ, et al. Young age is not a predictor of mortality in burns. Pediatr Crit Care Med 2001;2:223–4.
30. Ryan CM, Lee A, Kazis LE, et al. Multicenter Burn Outcome Group. Recovery trajectories after burn injury in young adults: does burn size matter? J Burn Care Res 2015;36:118–29.

Burn Resuscitation in the Austere Environment

Michael Peck, MD, ScD[a],*, James Jeng, MD[b], Amr Moghazy, MD, MSc, PhD[c]

KEYWORDS

- Burn shock • Resuscitation • Resource-limited settings

KEY POINTS

The following are the 2016 recommendations for burn shock resuscitation from the International Society for Burn Injuries Practice Guidelines for Burn Care.

- Adult patients with burns greater than 15% total burn surface area (TBSA) and pediatric patients with burns greater than 10% TBSA should be formally resuscitated with salt-containing fluids; requirements should be based on body weight and percentage burn.

- When intravenous fluid administration is practical, between 2 to 4 mL/kg body weight/burn surface area (%TBSA) should be administered within the first 24 hours after injury, with alertness to over-resuscitation. Even in these cases, oral fluid supplementation is encouraged within the first 6 hours.

- If only oral fluid administration is practical, drinking liquids (typical of the local diet) equivalent to 15% of the body weight each 24 hours is recommended for 2 days. Five-gram tablets of table salt (or the equivalent) must be ingested for each liter of oral fluids.

- When practical, monitor the adequacy of resuscitation by titrating salt-containing fluids. For adults, titrate provided fluids to the average patient's range of urine output, that is, 0.3 to 0.5 mL/kg/h; in children titrate to 1.0 mL/kg/h.

INTRODUCTION

Burn shock is a condition that follows thermal injury to the skin and is defined by inadequate oxygen delivery to organs and insufficient elimination of tissue metabolites. Burn shock, along with smoke inhalation injury, if not treated appropriately, is the most common cause of death after burn injury.

Intravenous (IV) administration of fluids is the gold standard for burn shock resuscitation. Electrolyte solutions such as lactated Ringer or Hartmann solution can effectively prevent or treat burn shock. Several formulas, some which advise the use of colloids within the first 24 hours, guide the clinician in establishing the proper rate of fluid administration; however, remain alert to over-resuscitation. Particularly in a

[a] Arizona Burn Center, Maricopa Medical Center, 2601 East Roosevelt Street, Phoenix, AZ 85008, USA; [b] Mount Sinai Healthcare System, New York, NY, USA; [c] Suez Canal University, Suez Canal University Hospitals, Ismailia, Egypt
* Corresponding author.
E-mail address: michael_peck@dmgaz.org

resource-limited setting (RLS), in the first 24 hours after burn injury, the use of crystalloid formulas, such as the Parkland or Brooke formula, ensures the rescue of the almost all burn survivors from burn shock in a cost-effective manner.

In a RLS, however, the supplies and equipment to administer large volumes of IV fluids may be deficient. Scarcities may include IV catheters and lines, a limited number of health care personnel trained in the administration of IV fluids, and a shortage of sterile IV fluids with the appropriate electrolyte composition. In addition, patients might take hours to reach a facility where IV administration is available. Therefore, in austere environments an alternative plan for fluid resuscitation is required for burn care.

Oral rehydration therapy (ORT) is a well-established technique for preventing dehydration caused by diarrhea in RLS.[1] Basically, ORT is the technique of giving patients adequate amounts of a solution containing glucose and electrolytes by mouth. ORT can be delivered at low cost by local health care workers or family members. For example, a child with diarrhea can be rehydrated using ORT at a cost of only US $0.67 (2015 cost estimates).[2,3]

Since 1975, the United Nations Children's Fund (UNICEF) and the World Health Organization (WHO) have provided packets of glucose and salts to be used in ORT for infectious diarrhea. The earliest formulation of this solution contained glucose, sodium chloride, potassium chloride, and trisodium citrate, with a resultant osmolarity of 311 mOsm/L. The formula was modified in 2003, and the current recommendations advise the use of oral rehydration salt solution (ORS) with reduced osmolarity to minimize stool output from diarrhea.[2,3]

Even though prospective, randomized clinical trials have not yet been conducted, expert opinion is that ORT can be effectively used to resuscitate patients from burn shock, provided that there are no other illnesses or injuries that would prevent safe oral intake and that the burn size is not unduly large.[4–7] Especially under circumstances in which the alternative is no resuscitation, the potential benefits from ORT outweigh the risks, such as hyponatremia.[8,9] According to Monafo,[10] high-salt fluids administered to burn patients reduced the needed volume for resuscitation compared with isotonic solutions. It might be more appropriate, therefore, to add salt supplement to the WHO-ORS solution, and administer that according to the Sørensen formula.[11]

Rectal infusion therapy (proctoclysis) is another tactic that may be helpful in remote or rural settings.[12] Proctoclysis was used for treatment of battlefield injuries in both world wars after its introduction by John Benjamin Murphy in the early twentieth century to treat shock from peritonitis.

PATIENT EVALUATION OVERVIEW

The gastrointestinal tract has the capacity to absorb large amounts of fluid, as much as 20 L per day.[13] The intestine retains its ability to absorb fluid notwithstanding the presence of burns of up to 40% TBSA.[5] Rectal infusions of either saline or tap water have been tolerated at rates up to 400 mL/h.[14]

Free (pure) water is potentially lethal to patients recovering from burn shock. Severe hyponatremia, as well as cerebral edema and death, may occur if patients are allowed to drink free water.[6] Sodium is, therefore, an absolute requirement in burn resuscitation using ORS.

Nutrient-independent salt-absorption exchange mechanisms, sodium/hydrogen (Na^+/H^+) and chlorine/bicarbonate (Cl^-/HCO_3^-), are present in enterocytes, but the sodium-glucose cotransporter (SGLT1) moves a significant portion of sodium from the intestinal lumen. For every molecule of glucose, 2 sodium ions are transported; thus, the osmolality of ORS can be increased and transport of sodium facilitated by addition of glucose polymers, rice powders, or other simple carbohydrates.[15]

PHARMACOLOGIC TREATMENT OPTIONS

With ORT, patients with up to 20% TBSA can be easily resuscitated, and some with burns of up to 40% TBSA can be resuscitated successfully. Up to 15% of the total resuscitation fluids can be given orally in the hospital if combined with IV fluids. If urine output is satisfactory, IV fluid can be decreased as long as ORT can be maintained. In the prehospital setting, the determination regarding the amount of ORT to administer is made by the availability or shortage of IV fluids and equipment. If oral intake is restricted, additional fluids and electrolytes can be given by proctoclysis.

The cost of ORT is a minor expense, even in a RLS. There are many options for ORT:

- ORS packets can be purchased commercially.
- To create ORS, use 1 L of clean water, one teaspoon of table salt (3 g), and 3 tablespoons of sugar (18 g or 9 sugar cubes). One salt tablet can be substituted for each teaspoon of table salt.
- To reduce water contamination, boil the water; or add chlorine drops, iodine tablets, or potassium alum.
- Baking soda (sodium bicarbonate), a source of sodium, can be used as an alternative to table salt.
- A worldwide list of commercial manufacturers and distributers of ORS products can be found at http://rehydrate.org/resources/suppliers.htm (Accessed January 11, 2016).
- If it is not possible to measure the quantity of added salt, the solution should have the taste of tears.
- Molasses and other forms of raw sugar can be substituted for white table sugar, although both brown sugar and molasses add additional potassium.
- If the water is boiled before adding ingredients, salt and sugar should be added while it is still warm. If the solution is boiled after the sugar has been added, it will decompose.
- The patient should be instructed to drink sips of approximately 50 mL every 5 minutes, with the goal of drinking at least 4 cups (1 L) per hour. If vomiting occurs, the patient should wait 10 minutes before attempting to drink again.
- Keep the solution cool if possible. After 24 hours the solution should be discarded and a new batch made.

Other options for ORT include

- Rice water (congee) with salt
- Fresh lime water with salt and sugar
- Vegetable or chicken soup with salt
- Lassi (yogurt drink with salt and sugar)
- Sugarcane juice with lemon, black pepper, and salt
- Sports drink (eg, Gatorade or Powerade) with one-fourth teaspoon salt and one-fourth teaspoon baking soda for each quart
- Carrot soup
- Gruel (cooked cereal diluted with water)
- Noncaffeinated soda drinks that have been allowed to decarbonate by going flat.

Drinks to be avoided include

- Carbonated soda drinks with high fructose corn syrup and caffeine
- Fruit drinks with high sugar content
- Sweet tea or coffee
- Herbal teas that contain diuretics.

Procedure for performing proctoclysis[12]

- Boil water to reduce risk of infection or allergic reaction
- Warm water to body temperature
- Create balanced rehydration solution by the addition of salt and bicarbonate as previously described
- Insert urethral catheter into rectum
- Attach reservoir (eg, 50 mL syringe with plunger removed) to catheter
- Infuse fluids at a rate comfortable to the patient and consistent with clinical signs.

EVALUATION OF OUTCOME AND LONG-TERM RECOMMENDATIONS

Years of clinical experience with burn shock resuscitation demonstrate that monitoring the adequacy of burn resuscitation efforts is of great consequence to outcomes.[16] The use of bladder catheters is not practical in RLS; they also lead to potential infectious consequences. However, the accuracy and applicability of using simpler methods, such as weighing diapers, to quantify urine output are not well documented. For the most part, monitoring of urine output during burn shock resuscitation is the most effective and efficacious approach to confirm adequate resuscitation. Thus, is it recommended that fluids be titrated to the range of average adult patients' urine outputs: 0.3 to 0.5 mL/kg/h; in children the endpoint should be 1.0 mL/kg/h. Another effective method of resuscitation is to collect the hourly specific gravity of the urine. To reduce cost, and adapt for the RLS and lower-income or middle-income countries, use of the simple hydrometer is recommended.

SUMMARY

Intravenous (IV) cannulation and sterile IV salt solutions may not be options in resource-limited settings (RLSs). This article presents recipes for fluid resuscitation in the aftermath of burns occurring in RLSs. Burns of 20% total body surface area (TBSA) can be resuscitated, and burns up to 40% TBSA can most likely be resuscitated, using oral resuscitation solutions (ORSs) with salt supplementation. Without IV therapy, fluid resuscitation for larger burns may only be possible with ORSs. Published global experience is limited, and the magnitude of burn injuries that successfully respond to World Health Organization ORSs is not well-described.

REFERENCES

1. World Health Organization, United Nations Children's Fund. Oral rehydration salts: production of the new ORS. Geneva (Switzerland): WHO Press; 2006. Available at: http://whqlibdoc.who.int/hq/2006/WHO_FCH_CAH_06.1.pdf. Accessed December 27, 2012.
2. United Nations Children's Fund. New formulation of oral rehydration salts (ORS) with reduced osmolarity. New York: UNICEF Press; 2014. Technical bulletin No. 9. Available at: http://www.unicef.org/supply/files/Oral_Rehydration_Salts%28ORS%29_.pdf. Accessed January 26, 2016.

3. United Nations Children's Fund, World Health Organization. Reduced osmolarity oral rehydration salts (ORS) formulation: a report from a meeting of experts jointly organized by UNICEF and WHO. Geneva (Switzerland): WHO Press; 2002. Available at: http://apps.who.int/iris/bitstream/10665/67322/1/WHO_FCH_CAH_01.22.pdf. Accessed December 27, 2012.

4. Cancio LC, Kramer GC, Hoskins SL. Gastrointestinal fluid resuscitation of thermally injured patients. J Burn Care Res 2006;27:561–9.

5. Michell MW, Oliveira HM, Kinsky MP, et al. Enteral resuscitation of burn shock using World Health Organization oral rehydration solution: a potential solution for mass casualty care. J Burn Care Res 2006;27:819–25.

6. Kramer GC, Michell MW, Oliveira H, et al. Oral and enteral resuscitation of burn shock—the historical record and implications for mass casualty care. Eplasty 2010;10:e56.

7. Milner SM, Greenough WB 3rd, Asuku ME, et al. From cholera to burns: a role for oral rehydration therapy. J Health Popul Nutr 2011;29:648–51.

8. Jeng J, Gibran N, Peck M. Burn care in disaster and other austere settings. Surg Clin North Am 2014;94:893–907.

9. El-Sonbaty MA. Oral rehydration therapy in moderately burned children. Annals of the Mediterranean Burn Club (MBC) 1991;4:29–32.

10. Monafo WW. The treatment of burn shock by the intravenous and oral administration of hypertonic lactated saline solution. J Trauma 1970;10:575–86.

11. Sørensen B. Saline solutions and dextran solutions in the treatment of burn shock. Ann N Y Acad Sci 1968;150:865–73.

12. Tremayne V. Emergency rectal infusion of fluid in rural or remote settings. Emerg Nurse 2010;17:26–8.

13. Sladen G. Methods of studying intestinal absorption in man. In: McColl I, Sladen G, editors. Intestinal absorption in man. London: Academic Press; 1975. p. 10–25.

14. Bruera E, Schoeller T, Pruvost M. Proctoclysis for hydration of terminal cancer patients. Lancet 1994;344:1699.

15. Duggan C, Fontaine O, Pierce NF, et al. Scientific rationale for a change in the composition of oral rehydration solution. JAMA 2004;291:2628–31.

16. Warden GD. Burn shock resuscitation. World J Surg 1992;16:16–23.

How to Recognize a Failed Burn Resuscitation

Elisha G. Brownson, MD[a], Tam N. Pham, MD[a],*, Kevin K. Chung, MD[b,c]

KEYWORDS

- Burn • Resuscitation • Failed • Difficult • Runaway • Morbidity • Death

KEY POINTS

- Failed resuscitation can be defined as one associated with major complications that do not allow the patient to progress to the next phase in care.
- Triggers and protocols may be used to aid in early identification of threatened failure of resuscitation.
- When failed resuscitation occurs, and futility of care arises, a transition to comfort care measures should be initiated.

INTRODUCTION

Massive burn injury results in a dysregulated host response characterized by widespread capillary leak resulting in volume redistribution, decreased tissue perfusion, and subsequent end-organ failure. There are many factors that may add to the magnitude of this response. The mainstay of therapy in the initial care of these patients includes the initiation of judicious intravenous fluids that are titrated in response to a compilation of various physiologic and laboratory endpoints, anchored on the close monitoring of urine output. Over the years, a lot of attention has been focused on over-resuscitation and the physiologic cost of overzealous fluid management.[1] Recently, the consequences of under-resuscitation have come into question.[2]

The authors have nothing to disclose.

Department of Defense Disclaimer: The opinions or assertions contained herein are the private views of the authors and are not to be construed as official or as reflecting the views of the Department of the Army or the Department of Defense. The views expressed herein are those of the authors and do not reflect the official policy or position of the US Army Institute of Surgical Research, the Department of the Army and Department of Defense, or the US government.

[a] Department of Surgery, Harborview Medical Center, 325 Ninth Avenue, Box 359796, Seattle, WA 98104, USA; [b] United States Army Institute of Surgical Research, 3698 Chambers Pass, JBSA Fort Sam Houston, TX 78234, USA; [c] Department of Surgery, Uniformed Services University of the Health Sciences, 4301 Jones Bridge Road, Bethesda, MD 20814, USA

* Corresponding author.

E-mail address: tpham94@uw.edu

Crit Care Clin 32 (2016) 567–575

http://dx.doi.org/10.1016/j.ccc.2016.06.006

0749-0704/16/$ – see front matter © 2016 Elsevier Inc. All rights reserved.

criticalcare.theclinics.com

Regardless, successful burn resuscitation is one that enables the patient to survive, with minimal morbidity, to the next phase of care, allowing for surgical intervention. Despite decades of experience with resuscitation, burn providers still encounter a small subset of patients who fare poorly during the resuscitation phase. Thus, a failed resuscitation can be defined as one associated with major complications that do not allow the patient to progress to the next phase in care. This article focuses entirely on this population.

RECOGNIZING A FAILED BURN RESUSCITATION

Perhaps the most important factor in avoiding a failed resuscitation is the early recognition of a difficult or runaway resuscitation by the burn care provider. An early recognition of the signs and symptoms of a threatened failed resuscitation will allow for prompt initiation of rescue therapies and the subsequent delineation of goals of care in nonresponders. The authors suggest 3 critical periods during burn resuscitation when failure can be declared (**Table 1**), each with distinct features that providers must recognize promptly. The authors propose early failure as the first 8 hours of hospitalization, in-resuscitation failure as 8 to 24 hours, and late failure as beyond 24 hours.

Table 1
Typical clinical signs of failing resuscitation, by time of onset

Category	Admission to First 8 h	Hours 8–24	Beyond 24 h
Resuscitation and hemodynamics	Multiple crystalloid infusion rate increases without adequate response Hypotension Vasopressor requirement	Ongoing fluid administration exceeds 1.5–2 times predicted fluid needs Need to increase crystalloid fluid rate after initial reduction attempt Inadequate or no response to colloid supplementation Hypotension Catecholamine-resistant shock (multiple vasopressors at rising doses)	Crystalloid fluid rate ≥300 mL/h Any increase in crystalloid fluid rate Inadequate or no response to colloid supplementation Hypotension Catecholamine resistant shock (multiple vasopressors at high doses)
Clinical impression	Oligouria/anuria	Oligouria/anuria Tight abdomen by physical examination	Oligouria/anuria Difficult to ventilate Deemed too unstable for operative eschar removal
Laboratory markers	Severe lactic acidosis	Hematocrit >>60% Hematocrit rises on serial checks Creatinine rise Persistent and severe metabolic acidosis, lactic acidosis, coagulopathy	Hematocrit >>50% Elevated creatinine Unresolved metabolic acidosis, lactic acidosis, coagulopathy

Burn care providers must have certain parameters by which to measure the success or failure of burn resuscitation. An honest and repeated reassessment of a patient's resuscitation trajectory will help recognize a runaway resuscitation instead of blindly accepting borderline results hour after hour until the resuscitation is not salvageable. Although thresholds are not clearly defined in the literature review, the authors propose several triggers that will alert the burn care provider of an imminent failed resuscitation. Often first signs will revolve around the deviation from the hourly fluid resuscitation estimates based on calculated predictive formulas. Signs of oliguria, hypotension, and worsening lactic acidosis despite increasing intravenous fluids should prompt the burn care provider to anticipate complications. The authors suggest that if the projected trajectory at any time during the resuscitation exceeds 250 mL/kg, it is likely that these overwhelming resuscitation needs will lead to a failed resuscitation.[3] Whereas laboratory markers may continue to worsen (eg, rising serum creatinine and worsening hemoconcentration) as the next indicators of potential failure, the patient will rapidly exhibit signs of circulatory shock and impending organ dysfunction. As the burn resuscitation continues past the initial 24-hour phase, the patient may transition into an unsalvageable state as ventilation difficulties may arise, catecholamine resistant shock ensues, and subsequent multiple organ failure sets in; this patient will ultimately fail to progress to the operative phase.

EARLY FAILURE OF RESUSCITATION

Early signs of failure will largely be determined by age and total body surface area (TBSA) burn injury size. Both extremes of age tend to not tolerate burn injury well; similarly, large TBSA burn size (>90%) may lead the burn care provider to determine that a burn resuscitation will be futile as the patient will not be able to survive the operative phase of care. Several predictive scoring systems have been used to aid providers in determining early failure. For instance, the revised Baux score has recently been proposed as a reliable predictor of mortality in the era of modern burn care.[4] Through analysis of recent results of the American Burn Association National Burn Repository (ABA-NBR), Osler and colleagues derived an estimate of percent mortality based on a nomogram that correlates with the sum of age + %TBSA burn + (17 × [inhalational injury: 1 = yes, 0 = no]). However, there are important caveats to consider. First, epidemiologic studies evaluate populations, whereas providers take care of individual patients. Thus limiting interventions based on an estimated percent mortality can be a difficult choice to make at the bedside. Nevertheless, the authors have observed (corroborated by the NBR) that survival to discharge becomes unlikely when the revised Baux score exceeds 130 to 140.[5] Second, mortality models often do not distinguish second-degree burns (may heal without surgery) versus third-degree areas (require operative intervention), or the severity of inhalation injury, as their accurate staging can be difficult on initial presentation. Finally, mortality prediction formulas often do not account for patient comorbidities, yet their contribution to mortality often outweighs the contribution from burns alone.[6] When evaluating a burn-injured patient on initial presentation, one must consider the patient's ability to survive all phases of care: resuscitative, operative, and rehabilitative. If the patient is not anticipated to survive and potentially rehabilitate, early transition to comfort care should be considered in order to avoid prolonging the patient's suffering unnecessarily.

Other signs of early burn failure will present as those patients who never meet standard resuscitation goals (eg, hypotension without pressors, lactic acidosis, or anuria despite multiple increases in crystalloid infusion) (see **Table 1**). Patients in this category have typically sustained massive skin burns in combination with severe inhalation injury. Many additional established and postulated risk factors may help predict a difficult resuscitation. These factors can be divided into patient, injury, provider/systems factors, as well as early complications (**Table 2**). Without proper recognition, early resuscitation failure often ensues. Thus, the burn provider faces difficult choices in early nonresponders, and should consider early initiation of available rescue therapies, even within the first 8 hours of resuscitation.[7]

IN-RESUSCITATION FAILURE

In-resuscitation failure may be difficult to determine, but these patients often present as nonresponders to rescue therapies. Initial resuscitation attempts will be fraught with increasing fluid needs, worsening laboratory values, hemodynamic instability, and worsening acidosis. As the potential for runaway burn resuscitation becomes evident, burn care providers may employ rescue strategies. Various adjunctive therapies exist (**Table 3**), with no clear consensus as to which therapies to employ.[8] The purpose of adjunctive therapies is to reduce crystalloid infusion rates and inflammatory burden, with the overarching goal of avoiding excessive volumes during the resuscitation phase.

The mainstay of initial rescue therapy is usually colloid infusion in the form of either albumin or plasma, which has been demonstrated to prevent or reverse the fluid

Table 2	
Factors that predict resuscitation failure	
Established Factors (with Broad Agreement)	**Postulated Factors (with Variable Clinical Evidence)**
Patient factors	
Prior dehydration	Hypoproteinemia
Alcohol and other drug intoxication	
Young pediatric patient	
Elderly patient	
Medical comorbidities	
Injury factors	
Very large TBSA cutaneous thermal burn	Admission hypothermia
Very deep cutaneous thermal burn	
Electrical burn	
Concomitant inhalation injury	
Cyanide toxicity	
Concomitant non-burn trauma	
Provider/systems factors	
Delay in initiation of resuscitation	Not using colloid as supplementation or rescue
Too high initial fluid rate	
Use of intravenous crystalloid boluses at initiation	Closed-circuit smart resuscitation
	Liberal or excessive use of pain/sedation infusions
Too high target goals for hemodynamics and urine output	Multiple patient hand-offs
Absence of strict fluid titration protocol	Provider inexperience
Poor adherence to fluid titration protocol	Delay in recognition (or acceptance) of acute kidney injury
Complications	
Vascular access complications	Gastrointestinal intolerance (to initiation of feedings)
Foley dislodgement/obstruction	
Acute kidney injury	

Table 3 Adjunctive therapies to intravenous fluid in burn resuscitation	
Adjunctive Therapy	**Postulated Mechanism**
Colloid infusion	
Albumin	Mitigates fluid creep and hypoalbuminemia
Plasma	Mitigates fluid creep
Plasma exchange	Reduces inflammatory burden
Hemofiltration	Blood purification; concurrently treats acute renal failure
Vitamin C	Antioxidant effect
Early burn eschar excision (within 24 h)	Reduces inflammatory burden

creep.[9–11] Other adjunctive therapies include plasma exchange,[12,13] high-dose vitamin C,[14] and early burn eschar excision.[15,16] Lack of sufficient Level 1 evidence for any of these maneuvers has greatly limited widespread adoption, and perhaps represents a significant barrier in advancing early burn care. Nevertheless, centers experienced in these rescue therapies report that they can mitigate or sometimes even prevent most runaway resuscitations.[8] Given the current state of knowledge, the authors contend that the importance of establishing strict protocol thresholds and initiating a rescue therapy probably outweighs the pros/cons of 1 rescue therapy over another. Data from resuscitations aided by computer decision strongly suggest the concept that strict monitoring, recognition, and early course correction help reduce total fluid administration.[17] Lack of response to any rescue maneuver alone, or in combination, also defines failed resuscitation. Despite all efforts, oliguria or anuria, refractory acidosis, and catecholamine resistant shock will continue to progress, and will predictably be accompanied by resuscitation-related morbidities, such as difficulty with ventilation or development of abdominal compartment syndrome.

LATE FAILURE OF RESUSCITATION

End-organ failure may be diagnosed during the course of burn resuscitation (**Table 4**) and is usually a sign of late failure. Many of these end-organ morbidities will be managed with supportive care. However, certain end-organ failures mandate procedural or operative intervention. Elevated compartment pressures of extremities[18] (both burned and non-burned), abdomen,[3,19] and intraocular[20] may require decompression. Intraabdominal compartment syndrome may be predominantly caused by bowel edema, or ascites. In the latter case, bedside peritoneal drainage catheter placement may be sufficient decompression as a temporizing measure.[21] Of course, all interventions should be considered in light of goals of care and likelihood of survival before proceeding.

Whereas certain procedures can be accomplished at the bedside, others may require transport to the operating room, depending on the personnel, equipment, and expertise. Burn surgeons have traditionally been hesitant to transport a critical burn patient to the operating room in the first 24 hours, in order to avoid further challenging their physiologic derangement with blood loss, major fluid shifts, hypothermia risk, and other complications. Thus, the common practice is to wait until fluid resuscitation is (or is nearly) completed. Yet, one must remember that the burn eschar presents a massive inflammatory burden that could be contributing to increased resuscitation requirements. In the setting of resuscitation failure, waiting for the resuscitation phase to end usually means death of the patient. Safe operative removal of

Table 4
End-organ morbidities as a consequence of failed resuscitation

Organ System	Manifestation(s), by Increasing Severity
Central nervous system	Altered mental status Brain edema Increased intraocular pressures
Respiratory	Airway edema (with urgent need for intubation) High peak and plateau ventilatory pressures Respiratory acidosis Hypoxia Pleural effusions Inability to ventilate
Cardiovascular	Severe tachycardia Hypotension Low cardiac output Bradycardia
Renal	Persistent metabolic acidosis Oligouria Red pigmented urine Rise in creatinine (and other markers)
Hepatic	Persistent lactic acidosis Liver enzyme elevation Coagulopathy Jaundice
Abdominal	Bowel wall edema New-onset ascites Intra-abdominal hypertension Abdominal compartment syndrome
Skin/integument	Severe anasarca Skin weeping Elevated compartment pressures, even in nonburned extremities Burn wound conversion

burn eschar within the first 24 hours has been anecdotally performed, and is currently debated. Surgeons and other injury providers have also learned from damage control strategies for blunt and penetrating trauma over the past 20 years that emphasize balanced resuscitation and limiting operative interventions.[22,23] With damage control protocols more prominent today, many institutions have reported improved outcomes after severe trauma.[24,25] These reports have now led to the extension of damage control strategies to emergency general surgery[26] and challenge burn providers to consider developing protocols and collaboration with anesthesia providers to operate safely on burn injuries in the first 24 hours. Ultra-early removal of the clearly demarcated full-thickness burn eschar in the first 24 hours to limit fluid resuscitation could be an application of damage control principles to burn surgery, thus constituting a paradigm shift in burn care.

Another consideration of end-organ dysfunction is when to accept some measure of organ failure in lieu of death. The provider must decide which organ failure to accept, and which can be recoverable in the setting of multiple organ dysfunction syndrome (MODS). The typical scenario is a patient who has developed anasarca, but remains oliguric or anuric with increased ventilatory requirements. As MODS persists, the overwhelming demands of these complications will stall resuscitation and indicate that this patient will not progress to the next phase of burn care. In this dire situation, the risks of continued over-resuscitation outweigh acceptance of acute kidney injury.[2] Instead of continuing on the same trajectory, providers may decide to reduce intravenous fluids to avert fluid overload, inability to ventilate, and certain death. Implementing continuous renal replacement therapy (CRRT) often mitigates severe electrolyte imbalance and continued third spacing sufficiently to bridge the patient to operative care. If the patient survives, full renal recovery is possible, especially in younger individuals. There is a subset of patients in whom end-organ dysfunction will persist and deteriorate, despite maximal efforts of the burn care provider. As late failed resuscitation declares itself, these patients will either proceed to death despite active care or will be transitioned to comfort care measures.

TRANSITIONING GOALS OF CARE

When a burn care provider is faced with a high likelihood of failed resuscitation, at any point in an injured patient's care, they must assess the futility of care and consider transitioning their goals of care to that of comfort to avoid propagation of suffering. Although this may be straightforward in some cases, many cases will be less clear, and resuscitation will continue as additional information is obtained.[27] In addition to premorbid medical conditions and variables that signal the likelihood of a failed resuscitation, one must consider views and wishes of the patient (ideally) or family (surrogate). When possible, a family conference is the best format to discuss and make goals of care decisions. Palliative care consultation has been advocated as an early intervention in the intensive care unit for patients with an overwhelming likelihood of death. However, the nature of burn injuries may necessitate that goals of care decisions be made expediently at all hours, and these conversations should not be delayed. Thus, the burn care provider must ultimately be the advocate to transition from resuscitative intent to a palliative intent when the patient's condition deteriorates to the point of non survivability.[28] Once palliation becomes the primary goal, burn providers must ensure symptom palliation (pain, distress) for the dying patient, while effectively stopping all life-sustaining therapies (fluids, pressor, nutrition, and finally ventilator support).[29] In addition, nurses and social workers have complementary roles in assisting with grief and bereavement support for the patient's family. Finally, a chaplain can often help address spiritual concerns of the patient and family.

SUMMARY

Burn care providers should be aware of patient and injury characteristics that may predispose the injured patient to a difficult resuscitation. As the burn resuscitation progresses, high fluid requirements, above calculated estimates, will trigger the provider to recognizing development of failure. As organ dysfunction develops, the provider will need to employ adjunctive rescue maneuvers and consider damage control burn surgery when applicable. Throughout each stage of the resuscitation, early identification and intervention may help convert a runaway resuscitation to a successful transition to the next phase of care. However, this must be counterbalanced with the prompt recognition of when the point of resuscitation failure has been reached. Recognition of and acceptance of futility are important first steps that can significantly impact the quality of end-of-life care in burns.

REFERENCES

1. Pruitt BA Jr. Protection from excessive resuscitation: "pushing the pendulum back". J Trauma 2000;49(3):567–8.

2. Mason SA, Nathens AB, Finnerty CC, et al, Inflammation and the Host Response to Injury Collaborative Research Program. Hold the pendulum: rates of acute kidney injury are increased in patients who receive resuscitation volumes less than predicted by the parkland equation. Ann Surg 2016. [Epub ahead of print].

3. Ivy ME, Atweh NA, Palmer J, et al. Intra-abdominal hypertension and abdominal compartment syndrome in burn patients. J Trauma 2000;49(3):387–91.

4. Osler T, Glance LG, Hosmer DW. Simplified estimates of the probability of death after burn injuries: extending and updating the Baux score. J Trauma 2010,68(3). 690–7.

5. Hodgman E, Joseph B, Mohler J, et al. Creation of a decision aid for goal setting after geriatric burns: a study from the prognostic assessment of life and limitations after trauma in the elderly [PALLIATE] consortium. J Trauma Acute Care Surg 2016;81:168–72.

6. Heng JS, Clancy O, Atkins J, et al. Revised Baux Score and updated Charlson comorbidity index are independently associated with mortality in burns intensive care patients. Burns 2015;41(7):1420–7.

7. Park SH, Hemmila MR, Wahl WL. Early albumin use improves mortality in difficult to resuscitate burn patients. J Trauma Acute Care Surg 2012;73(5):1294–7.

8. Bacomo FK, Chung KK. A primer on burn resuscitation. J Emerg Trauma Shock 2011;4(1):109–13.

9. Cartotto R, Callum J. A review of the use of human albumin in burn patients. J Burn Care Res 2012;33(6):702–17.

10. Lawrence A, Faraklas I, Watkins H, et al. Colloid administration normalizes resuscitation ratio and ameliorates "fluid creep". J Burn Care Res 2010;31(1):40–7.

11. O'Mara MS, Slater H, Goldfarb IW, et al. A prospective, randomized evaluation of intra-abdominal pressures with crystalloid and colloid resuscitation in burn patients. J Trauma 2005;58(5):1011–8.

12. Neff LP, Allman JM, Holmes JH. The use of therapeutic plasma exchange (TPE) in the setting of refractory burn shock. Burns 2010;36(3):372–8.

13. Mosier MJ, DeChristopher PJ, Gamelli RL. Use of therapeutic plasma exchange in the burn unit: a review of the literature. J Burn Care Res 2013;34(3):289–98.

14. Tanaka H, Matsuda T, Miyagantani Y, et al. Reduction of resuscitation fluid volumes in severely burned patients using ascorbic acid administration: a randomized, prospective study. Arch Surg 2000;135(3):326–31.

15. Chang KC, Ma H, Liao WC, et al. The optimal time for early burn wound excision to reduce pro-inflammatory cytokine production in a murine burn injury model. Burns 2010;36(7):1059–66.

16. Ong YS, Samuel M, Song C. Meta-analysis of early excision of burns. Burns 2006; 32(2):145–50.

17. Salinas J, Chung KK, Mann EA, et al. Computerized decision support system improves fluid resuscitation following severe burns: an original study. Crit Care Med 2011;39(9):2031–8.

18. Orgill DP, Piccolo N. Escharotomy and decompressive therapies in burns. J Burn Care Res 2009;30(5):759–68.

19. Hobson KG, Young KM, Ciraulo A, et al. Release of abdominal compartment syndrome improves survival in patients with burn injury. J Trauma 2002;53(6): 1129–33 [discussion: 1133–4].

20. Sullivan SR, Ahmadi AJ, Singh CN, et al. Elevated orbital pressure: another untoward effect of massive resuscitation after burn injury. J Trauma 2006;60(1):72–6.

21. Latenser BA, Kowal-Vern A, Kimball D, et al. A pilot study comparing percutaneous decompression with decompressive laparotomy for acute abdominal compartment syndrome in thermal injury. J Burn Care Rehabil 2002;23(3):190–5.
22. Ball CG. Damage control surgery. Curr Opin Crit Care 2015;21(6):538–43.
23. Shapiro MB, Jenkins DH, Schwab CW, et al. Damage control: collective review. J Trauma 2000;49(5):969–78.
24. Suen K, Skandarajah AR, Knowles B, et al. Changes in the management of liver trauma leading to reduced mortality: 15-year experience in a major trauma centre. ANZ J Surg 2015. [Epub ahead of print].
25. Rotondo MF, Schwab CW, McGonigal MD, et al. 'Damage control': an approach for improved survival in exsanguinating penetrating abdominal injury. J Trauma 1993;35(3):375–82 [discussion: 382–3].
26. Stawicki SP, Brooks A, Bilski T, et al. The concept of damage control: extending the paradigm to emergency general surgery. Injury 2008;39(1):93–101.
27. Cleland H. Death and the burn patient: who, how and when. Burns 2014;40(5):786–7.
28. Pham TN, Otto A, Young SR, et al. Early withdrawal of life support in severe burn injury. J Burn Care Res 2012;33(1):130–5.
29. Kelley AS, Morrison RS. Palliative care for the seriously III. N Engl J Med 2015;373(8):747–55.

Complicated Burn Resuscitation

David T. Harrington, MD, FACS

KEYWORDS

- Heart failure • Cirrhosis • Inhalation injury • Acute renal failure

KEY POINTS

- New technology and new information are helping improve the care of thermally injured patients during resuscitation.
- Reliance on old criteria and old-school judgment to guide resuscitation still has a role in management.
- There is an absolute combination of injury severity and lack of physiologic reserve that is uniformly fatal.

INTRODUCTION

More than 4 decades after the creation of the Brooke and Parkland formulas, burn practitioners still passionately argue about which formula is the best. So it is no surprise that there is a lack of consensus about the conundrum of trying to resuscitate a thermally injured patient with a significant comorbidity such as heart failure or cirrhosis or how to resuscitate a patient after an electrical or inhalation injury or a patient whose resuscitation is complicated by renal failure. To a large degree, all of these scenarios share a common theme in that the standard rule book does not apply. None of these patients can be resuscitated in a usual or standard fashion. All will require highly individualized resuscitations. There will be scenarios where advanced monitoring may be in the patient's best interest, and there are cases where careful titration of therapy to the old-school clinical signs of cardiac output—mental status, urine output and skin perfusion—may be ideal.

HEART FAILURE

A thermally injured patient with significant pre-existing heart failure is truly an acute on chronic failure problem. The baseline pathophysiology of the patient's cardiac disease is added to the hypovolemia and myocardial depression of an acute burn. Heart failure

Disclosure Statement: The author has nothing to disclose.
Rhode Island Burn Center, Rhode Island Hospital, Warren Alpert Medical School of Brown University, 593 Eddy Street, APC 444, Providence, RI 02903, USA
E-mail address: DHarrington@Lifespan.org

Crit Care Clin 32 (2016) 577–586
http://dx.doi.org/10.1016/j.ccc.2016.06.005
0749-0704/16/$ – see front matter © 2016 Elsevier Inc. All rights reserved.

is estimated to affect 2 to 3 million Americans, with a rate that significantly increases after the age of 45 and by the age of 65 affects men and women at equal rates.[1] The etiologies of heart failure are primarily ischemic, but also include mechanical dysfunction such as valvular disease and the nonischemic cardiomyopathies from viral, alcoholic, metabolic, and idiopathic causes. The clinical hallmarks of the failing myocardium are dysrhythmias, systolic dysfunction, and elevated diastolic tone. These manifestations of heart failure are driven by dysregulated calcium oscillations in the myocardium, resulting in high diastolic intracellular calcium and a remodeled heart where the myocardial architecture does not have the appropriate myocyte alignment secondary to the loss of the normal interstitial fibrillar collagen network. The failing heart provokes a neurohumoral response, such that resting sympathetic tone and baseline norepinephrine levels are elevated, and the renin-angiotensin-aldosterone axis is activated. Predictors of poor survival with heart failure are left ventricular (LV) ejection fraction less than 30%, LV end diastolic diameter greater than 7 cm, LV end diastolic volume (LVED) greater than 130 mL, serum norepinephrine greater than 600 pg/mL, narrow pulse pressure (systolic blood pressure, diastolic blood pressure [SBP-DBP/SBP <25%]) and New York Heart Association class 4 symptoms.

Burn injury unleashes a massive inflammatory cascade of histamine, prostaglandins, thromboxane, serotonin, catecholamines, and cytokines. These agents have the effect of reducing cardiac output and increasing systemic and pulmonary vascular resistance that is not corrected by normovolemia.[2–4] At baseline, the failing heart is living in an environment of increased sympathetic tone and stimulated neuroendocrine state, so an acute burn adds further to this stress and may identify some patients who have no further cardiac reserve. One of the strongest prognostic factors for survival in heart failure is whether patients respond to dobutamine. Patients who are maximally endogenously stimulated and who do not have any remaining functional reserve do not increase their cardiac output under dobutamine stimulation. These patients have a decreased rate of survival.[5] The stress of resuscitation may unmask these unfortunate patients early into their burn resuscitation.

Invasive monitoring of the heart by use of a Swan Ganz catheter, serial echocardiogram (ECHO) or other means is necessary for these brittle and often difficult-to-assess patients. The use of pulmonary artery (PA) catheters is declining in intensive care units due to concerns of insertion-related complications, potential infection risk, and data that suggest that the information obtained is not always used effectively. Initial enthusiasm for goal-directed therapy utilizing Swan-Ganz catheters to obtain ideal oxygen delivery and oxygen consumption endpoints has been dampened by the increased use of fluids needed for this strategy and the phenomenon of fluid creep seen in many burn centers in the last 15 years.[6] A survey of burn centers in Europe, the United States, Canada, and Australia showed that less than 8% of burn units use PA catheters frequently.[7] Unfortunately, the uncommon use of these catheters means that when the burn practitioner really needs these data (and in the heart failure patient undergoing acute burn resuscitation these data are critical), the team is less facile with obtaining and interpreting the data from the Swan-Ganz catheter. A new disposable minitransesophageal echocardiography device is now available that can be left in place for up to 72 hours. Initial use of this device has shown both safety and efficacy, but the costs are significant.[8,9] Serum B-type natriuretic peptide, a protein secreted from a stretched myocardium, has been shown to correlate with volume overload, and because it can be measured in a serial manner, it may be considered a way to screen for this state during resuscitation.[10] Careful volume resuscitation to restore adequate LVEDV and to keep right atrium pressure less than 8 and pulmonary artery occlusion pressure less than 18 is critical. In patients with a component of diastolic dysfunction, tolerate an even an even narrower range of LVED volume. Although there are no data on the use of angiotensin converting enzyme (ACE) inhibitors during acute resuscitation, there is strong evidence that ACE inhibitors are effective at off-loading the stress on the heart, and they should be restarted as soon as possible in these patients. Dobutamine, a β-1 agonist, and milrinone, a phosphodiesterase inhibitor, both act to increase cyclic –AMP intracellularly. Dobutamine should be started at 2.5 g/kg/min and titrated for effect. This drug can be arrhythmogenic, so monitoring for this occurrence is mandatory. Milrinone should be loaded at 50 g/kg over 20 minutes; then a maintenance dose of 0.375 to 0.75 g/kg/min is titrated to affect. Milrinone is associated with higher occurrence of hypotension than dobutamine and should not be used in states of relative hypovolemia. Milrinone also lowers pulmonary artery pressures, so it may be a good choice in patients with a component of pulmonary hypertension. Diuretics may be necessary for states of fluid overload, and a careful continuous infusion of diuretic will generally result in a more controlled and less labile swing in volume status as compared to intermittent bolus therapy. More advanced adjuncts to the failing myocardium in the presence of thermal injury are extrarenal fluid removal strategies as with continuous veno-venous hemodialysis (CVVH) and intra-aortic balloon counter pulsation (IABP). These strategies allow careful removal of fluid and minimize wide fluctuations in intravascular volume. IABP allows systolic afterload and augmented diastolic perfusion to the heart and brain. This device has significant limitations, in that the patient's mobility is severely restricted; there are downstream embolic events; and the devices can become infected. This therapy should only be entertained if there is a correctable cause of the myocardial dysfunction.

RENAL FAILURE

Up to 30% of severely thermally injured patients develop some degree of renal failure, with roughly one-third occurring in the first 5 days following burn, and most occurring later in the burn course, usually associated with sepsis.[11] The etiology of renal failure can be multifactorial. Hypovolemia and myocardial depression will result in hypoperfusion; systemic neurohumoral substances and cytokines can directly affect renal perfusion and cause direct renal parenchymal damage, and pigmenturia elaborated secondary to deep tissue injury can damage tubular cells and precipitate and occlude the renal tubular lumens. Prevention of renal failure involves ensuring adequate volume resuscitation, avoiding any nephrotoxic agents such as aminoglycosides, and treating pigmenturia if it occurs. Understanding, preventing, and managing acute renal failure are critical, for it is associated with an in-hospital mortality of 50% to 60% of critically-ill patients.[12]

How to ensure that the burn resuscitation is adequate is not easily determined, and how to determine whether 2 hours of anuria are the result of a stressed but still highly functioning kidney or the start of acute tubular necrosis (ATN) is equally difficult. The traditional hallmarks of a functioning kidney responding to an acute prerenal stress are a urine osmolality greater than 500, urine/plasma osmolality ratio greater than 2, a urinary sodium less than 20 mEq/L, and a fractional excretion of sodium less than 1 ($FE_{Na} = [U_{Na}/P_{Na}]/[U_{Cr}/P_{Cr}]$). The inability of the kidney to maintain these levels and the presence of renal tubular epithelial cells and granular casts in the urine are signs of ATN. Newer markers that are elevated in the presence of ATN are neutrophil gelatinase-associated lipocalin (NGAL), kidney injury marker 1 (KIM-1), N-acetyl-β-D-glucosaminidase (NAG), cystatin C, and interleukin (IL)-18. These markers can be measured in both the plasma and the urine, but the discriminatory power of the urinary markers is improved if their levels are indexed to urinary creatinine.[13,14] Although these markers can be helpful, their area under the curve values are 0.65 to 0.75; therefore elevation of these markers is not definitive, and they should be considered just another data point in making the diagnosis of ATN. These plasma and urinary tests do not outperform clinical criteria such as risk, injury, failure, loss of kidney function, and end-stage kidney disease (RIFLE) or Acute Kidney Injury Network (AKIN) clinical criteria in the first 24 hours after the onset of symptoms in the prognosis (days until recovery of renal function or rate of end-stage renal loss) of the acute renal failure event.[15]

Once the practitioner has determined that urine output is no longer a reliable marker of intravascular volume, there are 3 clinical decisions that need to be solved: how to measure intravascular volume and proceed with resuscitation; how to monitor and treat the complications of renal failure; and the timing and type of dialysis that may be needed. When considering how to monitor intravascular volume, it is important to realize that in the classification of hypovolemic shock, the signs of progression from Class 2 to Class 3 shock are the development of oliguria, the development of hypotension (SBP <90), and the start of agitation and confusion. A good burn resuscitation lives in this border between Class 2 and Class 3 shock. Too little fluid can cause renal failure, but too much fluid can result in the fluid overload and start the process of fluid creep that was seen in many burn centers in the last 15 years. The loss of urine output as a marker of volume still leaves blood pressure and mental status as reasonable arbiters of volume that can be used to titrate resuscitative fluid. Many practitioners will be uncomfortable with this limited knowledge. In this setting, the use of a Swan-Ganz catheter or other device can be useful. The treatment of the complication of renal failure is fairly straightforward. Once reasonable the diagnosis of ATN is certain, an attempt at converting oliguric renal failure to nonoliguric renal failure with the use of intravenous diuretics is warranted (furosemide 200 mg every 12 hours or furosemide 10–20 mg/h continuous infusion). Although there is no evidence that this will reduce the need for dialysis or result in earlier recovery of renal function, this may make the management of intravascular volume status easier and prevent the hypoxia associated with pulmonary congestion and edema. The development of hyperkalemia should be monitored with serum testing and cardiac monitoring (spiked T waves, flattening of P waves, and widened QRS complex). Significant hyperkalemia (K+ >6 or electrocardiogram [EKG] changes) should be treated with 500 mL of 10% dextrose and 20 units of regular insulin. Other treatments to reduce acidosis with sodium bicarbonate and delivery of calcium chloride should also be considered. Finally, some patients will need dialysis. Traditionally, the indications for dialysis are blood urea nitrogen (BUN) greater than 70 mg/dL, creatinine greater than 5 mg/dL, K+ greater than 6 mEq/L, base excess less than 15 mEq/L, pulmonary edema, or systemic uremic symptoms. Patients who meet these criteria should be dialyzed with either intermittent hemodialysis, in those patients with stable blood pressure, or with CVVH, in patients whose marginal intravascular volume status cannot tolerate the flow rates and the fluid withdrawal rates of intermittent dialysis without significant hypotension. With the proliferation of renal replacement machines in intensive care units (ICUs), there has been an interest in reassessing the traditional criteria for dialysis and exploring whether renal replacement therapy (RRT) early in a course of ATN will result in renal protection and earlier return of renal function that is not seen in traditional intermittent hemodialysis. Two recent randomized trials on this topic published in *The Journal of the American Medical Association* (JAMA) and *The New England Journal of Medicine* (NEJM) the same week have drawn different conclusions. The JAMA trial randomized patients to immediate start of RRT versus a wait and see initiation for RRT based on predefined criteria. The JAMA trial showed early initiation of RRT was associated with higher rates of return of renal function at 90 days (early 53.6%, late 38.7%, $P = .02$) and improved 90-day mortality (early 39.3%, late 54.7%, $P = .03$). Only 10% of the wait and see/delayed group avoided RRT.[16] The NEJM trial also randomized patients to immediate start of RRT versus a wait and see initiation for RRT. This trial showed an earlier return of spontaneous diuresis, lower rates of blood stream infections, and the avoidance of RRT in nearly half of the wait and see/delayed RRT group. They found no difference in mortality (early 48.5%, late 49.7%, $P = .79$).[17] Unfortunately, these trials, which randomized a total of 830 patients, have not given the burn practitioner a clear answer as to the appropriate timing of RRT for burn patients with ATN. Individual judgment of each patient's status is still needed.

CIRRHOSIS

In the setting of thermal injury, patients with cirrhosis are even more challenging than patients with heart failure. These cirrhotic patients are sometimes so far advanced in their disease that they literally have no physiologic reserve left. Add to that compromised status an acute burn resuscitation, and the burn practitioner has a tremendous clinical challenge.

Cirrhosis can be caused by toxin exposure (alcohol), viruses, prolonged cholestasis, autoimmune states (lupoid hepatitis), and metabolic diseases (alpha1-antitrypsin, hemochromatosis, Wilson). No matter the etiology of cirrhosis, the response to these injuries, hepatic necrosis followed by fibrosis and nodular regeneration, defines cirrhosis. Autopsy series show that cirrhosis exists in 3% to 5% of the US population. Many of these patients will not carry the diagnosis of cirrhosis upon admission to the burn center, but a careful history and physical examination or an elevated prothrombin time and a low albumin will alert the practitioner to the possibility of this condition. Ultrasound evaluation of the abdomen is useful to detect both a shrunken and irregular liver and potentially a large spleen. Early recognition is critical for the sequelae of cirrhosis, hepatocellular failure, and portal hypertension, which will severely complicate resuscitation. Hepatic blood flow averages 1500 mL/min and is approximately 25% of cardiac output. The 2 blood supplies to the liver, the portal vein and the hepatic artery, are regulated by different mechanisms. The portal blood supply is regulated indirectly by vasodilation/vasoconstriction of the splanchnic circulation, and the hepatic artery is regulated by sympathetic tone and circulating catecholamines. The scarring and regenerative nodules of cirrhosis create portal hypertension and make liver perfusion extremely sensitive to volume status. Hypovolemia can quickly result in further hepatocellular ischemia and necrosis. However, over-resuscitation with crystalloid can create tense ascites, which can further complicate resuscitation by loss of intravascular volume and intra-abdominal hypertension.

Cirrhosis has been shown to negatively impact outcomes in both blunt trauma and burns. In patients with blunt liver trauma, patients with cirrhosis had a rate of mortality quadruple the noncirrhotic patients (28% vs 7%), and this mortality difference widened if a laparotomy was required (58% vs 17%).[18] In the blunt trauma experience, the relative risk of mortality from cirrhosis can be predicted with the use of the model for end-stage liver disease (MELD) score. MELD is calculated using bilirubin, international normalized ratio (INR) and creatinine (MELD = 10 * [0.957 * ln(Creatinine)] + [0.378 * ln(Bilirubin)] + [1.12 * ln(INR)] + 6.43). Utilizing a receiver–operator analysis in blunt abdominal trauma, a MELD score of at least 17 was found to be the best predictor of a poor outcome for laparotomy.[19] Other authors have shown that each unit elevation of MELD increased the odds of mortality by 18%.[20] In thermally injured patients, the MELD score has not shown the same predictive power, but an analysis of the United States Army Institute of Surgical Research Burn Center showed a strong association of the diagnosis of cirrhosis with mortality. In patients with burn sizes between 10% and 50%, noncirrhotic patients had 12.7% mortality, but patients with cirrhosis had 83.3% mortality (P<.001).[21]

Patients with cirrhosis often have depleted levels of Factors V, VII, X potential from both malnutrition and decreased hepatic synthesis. Treatment with vitamin K and transfusion of fresh frozen plasma (FFP) is necessary in these patients. With advanced disease, there can also be an impairment of gluconeogenesis, which should be monitored for and treated with 10% glucose infusions. Resuscitating a patient with cirrhosis is the definition of walking a fine line, for neither mild hypervolemia nor hypervolemia is tolerated in these patients. An albumin- or FFP-based resuscitation is required, with less reliance on a standard crystalloid resuscitation. Early use of a Swan-Ganz catheter is helpful, but the practitioner should be aware that patients with cirrhosis will have a septic hemodynamic appearance when a Swan-Ganz catheter is used. The increased cardiac output and reduced systemic vascular resistance are most likely due to gut hormones and a reduced sensitivity of the splanchnic vasculature to catecholamines.[22] For these patients, cardiac output, mixed-venous O2 saturations, and SVR will be unreliable, leaving right atrial pressures and pulmonary artery occlusion pressures as the most reliable data to guide resuscitation.

ELECTRICAL INJURY

Electrical injury comprises only 3.5% of burn center admissions, but can have devastating effects. Electrical injury is the sixth leading cause of occupational deaths, representing 4.7% of all occupation-related deaths.[23] Electrical injuries can create 3 patterns of injury. The first is a true current injury, where the skin has been breached, and current passes through tissue, creating a path of predominately heat-related injury, although a nonheat injury, electroporation, also occurs in this type of injury.[24] The second type of electrical injury is an arc injury, which occurs when working in close proximity to electricity but without contact. Temperatures of electrical arcs can attain temperatures of 4000°C and result in a flash burn.[25] The last type is an electrical current that causes ignition of clothing or local aerosolized debris. The pattern of this injury is also a flash flame burn. Injuries from arcs and flash pattern injuries are treated just like standard cutaneous injuries and will not be discussed in this section. Injuries that involve over 1000 V, described as high voltage, are more likely to create the first type of injury, a true current injury. This type of injury can complicate burn resuscitation in many ways.

A true current injury that is most commonly caused by alternating current can create situations where patients are thrown from the electrical source. In these patients, a careful work-up for blunt trauma injuries is necessary, for rates of blunt injury can be as high as 15%. These injuries can also cause injury to the heart manifested by arrhythmias.[26] All patients with true current injury should have an admission EKG and cardiac monitoring for 24 hours if the admission EKG is abnormal. Often patients have only small areas of cutaneous injury, and much of the tissue injury is hidden underneath normal-appearing skin. The use of standardized resuscitation formulas will not be of much value. Starting patients at a 2 to 3 times maintenance fluid rate with lactated Ringer solution and then titrating to a urine output of 0.5 cc/kg/h is generally a safe and efficacious way to maintain an adequate intravascular volume. These patients may develop pigmenturia, which poses a significant threat to the kidneys from the precipitation of myoglobin and hemoglobin in the tubules, which can injure the tubular cells directly and can cause a mechanical obstruction of the tubules. Microscopic pigmenturia poses little risk to the patient, but a visible pigmenturia should be treated promptly. Two ampules of mannitol (ampule = 50 mL, 25%) is delivered via intravenous push (IVP) followed by 2 ampules (ampule = 50 mL, 1 meq/mL) of sodium bicarbonate via IVP. This therapy usually provokes an adequate urine output, and resuscitation can proceed normally. Further mannitol and bicarbonate are usually not necessary.[27] Following this treatment, continued careful monitoring of fluid status and maintaining adequate intravascular volume are critical. ATN following this injury is dependent on both the dose of the underlying muscle injury and presence of hypovolemia.[28] The edema from the electric current can cause compartment syndrome in all compartments along the current's path. Although prophylactic fasciotomies are not indicated, all compartments that show sign of compartment syndrome (distal pain, paresthesias, poikilothermia, pallor, lack of pulse) or elevated compartmental pressures should be decompressed promptly. Allowing a tense compartment to continue to elaborate components of muscle breakdown puts an unnecessary burden on the kidney to clear them.

INHALATION INJURY

Inhalation of smoke from a fire environment exposes the airways and the lungs to both a heat and chemical injury and occurs in almost 25% of thermally injured patients. The heat exposure is borne by the upper airways, the mouth, and pharynx in a vast majority of patients. Although this can result in upper airway edema and need for placement of an endotracheal tube, this injury should have little impact on resuscitation. The chemical injury from substances such as acrolein and formaldehyde are deposited to airways as fumes, mists, and/or aerosols deposited on soot. These and other chemicals provoke an immediate response in the airways, vasodilation of the bronchial artery and damage to the respiratory epithelium. Edema and bronchospasm of the conducting airways follow. Subsequently, there is development of a profound and diffuse exudative response from desquamated cells, lymph leak, and acute inflammatory cellular response that can occlude airways and lead to air trapping and ventilation-perfusion mismatch. In patients with combined cutaneous injury and inhalation injury, there is a reperfusion injury to the lung during the systemic ischemia reperfusion injury associated with burn resuscitation.[29] Although most of the 50 to 100 square meters of lung surface area are in the respiratory component, there is a significant surface area of the conducting airways. These conducting airways receive the largest amount of the chemical injury of inhalation injury, and this internal injury adds to the resuscitative fluid needs and increases the total amount of host injury.

Inhalation injury has been shown to add to the mortality following thermal injury with its impact at the middle range of burn acuity. One explanation for this increase in mortality is the added need for resuscitation volumes and higher rates of over-resuscitation driven by the additional injury to the lung surfaces.[30] Inhalation has been calculated to add 1.78 cc/kg/TBSA of fluid and 0.26 mEq/kg/TBSA of Na+ in the first 24-hour resuscitation.[31] The second reason inhalation injury impacts survival is the pulmonary dysfunction, need for mechanical ventilation, and the secondary pneumonias that develop in these patients.

Resuscitation of the patient with inhalation injury is perhaps the easiest of the dilemmas that have so far been reviewed in this article. The treatment of Carbon monoxide (CO) and Cyanide (CN) poisonings is straightforward. Although these 2 toxins affect oxygen delivery to the tissues by different mechanisms, the affect is the same: tissue hypoxia. In the setting of burn resuscitation and systemic ischemia, reperfusion further hypoxia should be avoided. One hundred percent oxygen should be delivered to patients with suspected and confirmed CO poisoning until the levels are less than 10%. One hundred percent oxygen reduces the half-life of CO from 250 minutes to 40 to 60 minutes as compared to room air. Most authors feel there is little role for hyperbaric oxygen in the treatment of CO poisoning. Although there is a further reduction of CO's half-life to 30 minutes with this therapy, most patients can have their CO reduced to nontoxic levels by the time the patient can be safely treated in a hyperbaric center; there are no good quality data that this therapy improves outcomes, and there is some risk to patient and attendants in a hyperbaric chamber.[32] In patients with cyanide levels greater than 20 ppm or signs of CN toxicity in patients who are suspected of having cyanide poisoning, such as unexplained mental status changes, myocardial ischemia, or lactic acidosis, treatment should start early. The first-line therapies should either be hydroxocobalamin (4 g) or sodium thiosulfate (125–250 mg/kg), which provides temporary and safe cyanide sinks so that the body can clear the toxin safely. Other treatments, such as nitrate administration, which oxidizes hemoglobin to methemoglobin and creates a cyanide sink, can create their own significant hazards to oxygen delivery. Luckily, nitrate therapy for CN toxicity is now only of historical interest. In terms of fluid resuscitation, the practitioner should not be surprised by the increased fluid needs of the patient with a combined cutaneous burn and pulmonary inhalation injury. With this understanding, careful and judicious fluid delivery is the course of therapy. The need for mechanical ventilation should be carefully considered. In the era of fluid creep, the recognition that more patients were receiving mechanical ventilation was discovered. This was felt to be a reflection of many prehospital protocols that overemphasized airway control for suspected inhalation injury.[33] However, the use of positive pressure ventilation decreases venous return to the heart by simply increasing intrathoracic pressure and affecting the feedback loop of the heart baroreceptors to reduce circulating blood volume.[34] Intubation is a therapeutic intervention with both good and bad clinical impact. Patients should only be intubated who truly need to be intubated, and, if intubated, ventilated with the lowest airway pressures possible during the sensitive 24- to 48-hour acute resuscitative period.

SUMMARY

Acute burn resuscitation continues to evolve. Patients with significant pre-existing heart failure should have adjuncts such as a Swan-Ganz catheter, a continuous ECHO device, or other devices to guide their resuscitation. The management of renal failure during acute burn resuscitation shows promise in that new markers of acute renal injury and new aggressive therapies such as CVVH may have a role of preserving renal function. There is much more to be learned about these modalities, and there is yet no true consensus on how these new technologies are best to be used. Patients with a significant burn and pre-existing cirrhosis pose an almost impossible clinical conundrum with extremely high rates of mortality despite maximal therapy. There does not appear to be anything on the horizon to change this sobering fact. Electrical injury poses many risks to the patient during, acute burn resuscitation, but careful time-honored treatments are still the mainstay of treatment. Inhalation injury is associated with increased volume and Na + requirements in the resuscitative period. In addition to careful titration of fluids, minimizing the impact of positive pressure ventilation during this critical resuscitation period is critical.

REFERENCES

1. National Center for Health Statistics. Health, United States 1990. U.S. Department of Health and Human Services. DHHS Publication No. (PHS) 91-1232. Washington, DC: U.S. Government Printing Office; 1991.

2. Horton JW, Garcia NM, White DJ, et al. Postburn cardiac contractile function and biochemical markers of postburn cardiac injury. J AM Coll Surg 1995;181(4): 289–98.

3. Horton JW, White J, Maass D, et al. Argininine in burn injury improves cardiac performance and prevents bacterial translocation. J Appl Physiol (1985) 1998;84(2): 695–702.

4. White J, Maass DL, Giroir B, et al. Development of an acute burn model in adult mice for studies of cardiac function and cardiomyocyte cellular function. Shock 2001;16(2):122–9.

5. Dubois-Rande JL, Merlet P, Roudot F, et al. Beta adrenergic contractile reserve as a predictor of clinical outcome in patients with idiopathic dilated cardiomyopathy. Am Heart J 1992;124(3):679–85.

6. Barton RG, Saffle JR, Morris SE, et al. Resuscitation of thermally injured patients with oxygen transport criteria as goals of therapy. J Burn Care Rehabil 1997;18(1 Pt 1):1–9.

7. Mansfield MD, Kinsella J. Use of invasive cardiovascular monitoring in patients with burns greater than 30 per cent body surface area: a survey of 251 centres. Burns 1996;22(7):549–51.

8. Fletcher N, Geisen M, Meeran H, et al. Initial clinical experience with a miniaturized transesophageal echocardiography probe in a cardiac intensive care unit. J Cardiothorac Vasc Anesth 2015;29(3):582–7.

9. Held JM, Litt J, Kennedy JD, et al. Surgeon-performed hemodynamic transesophageal echocardiography in the burn intensive care unit. J Burn Care Res 2016;37(1):e63–8.

10. Friese RS, Dineen S, Jennings A, et al. Serum B-type natriuretic peptide: a marker of fluid resuscitation after injury? J Trauma 2007;62(6):1346–50.

11. Holm C, Horbrand F, von Donnersmarck GH, et al. Acute renal failure in severely burned patients. Burns 1999;25(2):171–8.

12. Uchino S, Kellum JA, Bellomo R, et al. Acute renal failure in critically ill patients: a multinational, multicenter study. JAMA 2005;294(7):813–8.

13. Schley G, Köberle C, Manuilova E, et al. Comparison of plasma and urine biomarker performance in acute kidney injury. James LR, ed. PLoS One 2015; 10(12):e0145042.

14. Vaidya VS, Ferguson MA, Bonventre JV. Biomarkers of acute kidney injury. Annu Rev Pharmacol Toxicol 2008;48:463–93.

15. Koyner JL, Garg AX, Thiessen-Philbrook H, et al. Adjudication of etiology of acute kidney injury: experience from the TRIBE-AKI multi-center study. BMC Nephrol 2014;15:105.

16. Zarbock A, Kellum JA, Schmidt C, et al. Effect of early vs delayed initiation of renal replacement therapy on mortality in critically ill patients with acute kidney injury: the ELAIN Randomized Clinical Trial. JAMA 2016;315(20):2190–9.

17. Gaudry S, Hajage D, Schortgen F, et al. Initiation strategies for renal-replacement therapy in the intensive care unit. N Engl J Med 2016. http://dx.doi.org/10.1056/ NEJMoa1603017.

18. Barmparas G, Cooper Z, Ley EJ, et al. The effect of cirrhosis on the risk for failure of nonoperative management of blunt liver injuries. Surgery 2015;158(6): 1676–85.

19. Lin BC, Fang JF, Wong YC, et al. Management of cirrhotic patients with blunt abdominal trauma: analysis of risk factor of postoperative death with the model for End-Stage Liver Disease score. Injury 2012;43(9):1457–61.

20. Inaba K, Barmparas G, Resnick S, et al. The model for End-stage Liver Disease Score: an independent prognostic factor of mortality in injured cirrhotic patients. Arch Surg 2011;146(9):1074–8.
21. Burns CJ, Chung KK, Aden JK, et al. High risk but not always lethal: the effect of cirrhosis on thermally injured adults. J Burn Care Res 2013;34(1):115–9.
22. Benoit JN, Granger DN. Splanchnic hemodynamics in chronic portal hypertension. Semin Liver Dis 1986;6(4):287–98.
23. Cawley J, Homce G. Trends in Electrical Injury in the U.S., 1992-2002. 2006 Record of Conference Papers - IEEE Industry Applications Society 53rd Annual Petroleum and Chemical Industry Conference. 2006. 1–14. Available at: http:www.cdc.gov/niosh/mining/userfiles/works/pdfs/tieii.pdf.
24. Lee RC. Injury by electrical forces: pathophysiology, manifestations, and therapy. Curr Probl Surg 1997;34(9):677–764.
25. Nichter L, Bryant C, Kenny J, et al. Injuries due to commercial electric current. J Burn Care Rehabil 1984;5:124–37.
26. Housinger TA, Green L, Shahangian S, et al. A prospective study of myocardial damage in electrical injuries. J Trauma 1985;25(2):122–4.
27. Arnoldo BD, Purdue GF, Kowalske K, et al. Electrical injuries: a 20-year review. J Burn Care Rehabil 2004;25(6):479–84.
28. Sinert R, Kohl L, Rainone T, et al. Exercise-induced rhabdomyolysis. Ann Emerg Med 1994;23(6):1301–6.
29. Morris SE, Navaratnam N, Townsend CM Jr, et al. Bacterial translocation and mesenteric blood flow in a large animal model after cutaneous thermal and smoke inhalation injury. Surg Forum 1988;39:189–90.
30. Blumetti J, Hunt JL, Arnoldo BD, et al. The Parkland formula under fire: is the criticism justified? J Burn Care Res 2008;29(1):180–6.
31. Navar PD, Saffle JR, Warden GD. Effect of inhalation injury on fluid resuscitation requirements after thermal injury. Am J Surg 1985;150(6):716–20.
32. Grube BJ, Marvin JA, Heimbach DM. Therapeutic hyperbaric oxygen: help or hindrance in burn patients with carbon monoxide poisoning? J Burn Care Rehabil 1988;9(3):249–52.
33. Mackie DP, van Dehn F, Knape P, et al. Increase in early mechanical ventilation in burn patients: an effect of current emergency trauma management? J Trauma 2011;70(3):611–5.
34. Cancio LC, Chavez S, Alvarado-Ortega M, et al. Predicting increased fluid requirements during the resuscitation of thermally injured patients. J Trauma 2004;56(2):404–13.

Fluid Creep and Over-resuscitation

Jeffrey R. Saffle, MD

KEYWORDS

- Burns • Fluid resuscitation • Fluid creep • Colloid

KEY POINTS

- Fluid creep occurs when a patient requires more resuscitation fluid than is predicted by standard formulas.
- Fluid creep is reported in 30% to 90% of patients with major burns; the incidence increases with burn size.
- Excessive fluid given in the initial hours after injury predisposes to fluid creep.
- Complications of fluid creep include extremity and abdominal compartment syndromes, respiratory failure, and ocular hypertension. Resuscitations that require 6 mL/kg/% total body surface area or a total fluid of 250 mL/kg should prompt measures to correct fluid creep.
- Strategies to prevent or treat fluid creep include careful budgeting of fluids, use of colloid as a routine or rescue, hypertonic saline resuscitation, vitamin C infusions, and plasmapheresis.

INTRODUCTION

In 2000, Dr Basil Pruitt[1] coined the term fluid creep to characterize recent disturbing reports that many burn patients were receiving much more resuscitation fluid than predicted by widely accepted formulas. Not coincidentally, this insidious trend was preceded by widespread reports of the abdominal compartment syndrome (ACS)[2] and other serious complications. Pruitt called for clinicians to "push the pendulum back" by reassessing their resuscitation practices.

Reports of fluid creep have been widespread[3–23]; in response, clinicians have reexamined both the physiologic basis of burn shock and the historical underpinnings of revered resuscitation guidelines. The result has been enhanced appreciation of the complexities of burn resuscitation and several approaches for managing difficult patients through the critical period of initial burn treatment.

The author has no commercial or financial conflicts of interest with any product or individual mentioned in this article.
University of Utah Health Center, PO Box 102, Lake Elmo, MN 55042, USA
E-mail address: Jeffrey.saffle@me.com

Crit Care Clin 32 (2016) 587–598
http://dx.doi.org/10.1016/j.ccc.2016.06.007
criticalcare.theclinics.com

HISTORICAL CONTEXT

Clinicians have recognized and treated burn shock for almost a century. As experience and knowledge accumulated, progressively better formulas for fluid resuscitation were developed that dramatically reduced early burn mortality. Formula-guided resuscitation is now a cornerstone of modern care and the formulas themselves have become almost sacrosanct in the burn community. Foremost among these is Baxter's[4] Parkland formula, which originally called for lactated Ringer (LR) solution at a total dose of 4 mL/kg/% total body surface area (TBSA) burned, half given in the first 8 hours after injury, the rest over the next 16 hours. Importantly, he also emphasized that an infusion of plasma given during a fourth 8-hour period was essential to restore extracellular fluid volume and cardiac output. He reported that more than 79% of adults and 98% of children were successfully resuscitated with 3.7 to 4.3 mL/kg/% TBSA of LR. The earlier Brooke and Evans formulas also called for combinations of crystalloid and colloid.[24]

As these formulas became widely used, they were simplified and, ultimately, oversimplified. In 1979, the recommendations of a conference sponsored by the National Institutes of Health on burn care blended the crystalloid requirements of the most popular formulas, calling for initial resuscitation with LR at a total dose of 2 to 4 mL/kg/% TBSA, titrated to maintain urine output of 30 to 50 mL per hour, and omitting any routine use of colloids.[25] This became the consensus for burn resuscitation for over 25 years, and probably set the stage for the occurrence of fluid creep.

FLUID CREEP BEGINS

The Parkland formula was largely effective but not universally so. Even in the original reports, patient groups were noted who regularly required increased fluid volumes. Foremost among these were patients with inhalation injuries or high-voltage electrical injuries, and those in whom resuscitation was delayed. Subsequently, patients suffering multiple traumatic injuries, and those with acute alcohol or drug use, have been recognized to need extra fluid.[26]

Table 1 summarizes several clinical reports of burn resuscitation in a variety of circumstances. Several initial studies confirmed that fluid requirements were increased from 37% to 65% in the presence of inhalation injury, even with the addition of colloid.[27]

Fluid Creep: The New Normal?

In contrast to specific situations such as inhalation injury, more recent reports have described fluid creep in 30% to more than 80% of unselected patients without known complicating conditions. In many of these patients, fluid creep has a characteristic presentation: a patient arrives at the burn center having received substantially more crystalloid than required. Parkland resuscitation is begun and continues fairly smoothly until 8 to 12 hours after the burn injury. At that time, instead of decreasing, fluid requirements actually begin to escalate, ranging further and further from predictions. As this continues, problems with edema-related complications may become more obvious. Requirements for large quantities of crystalloid may continue unchecked despite efforts to reduce them and taper only very slowly, often requiring more than 24 hours to resolve.

As noted by Pruitt[1], the magnitude and frequency of this scenario seems to be a distinctly modern problem. Friedrich and colleagues[14] compared a small group of patients treated during 2000 with similar patients treated 25 years earlier and found that resuscitation requirements had doubled.[15] As possible explanations, the investigators

Table 1
Reports on fluid requirements in burn resuscitation

Author, Year	Number of Subjects[a]	Resuscitation Received (mL/kg/% TBSA)[b]	Comments
Baxter,[4] 1978	954	3.7–4.3	Original report of the Parkland formula 70% of 438 adults and 98% of 516 children resuscitated successfully with the volumes listed
Inhalation injury			
Baxter,[5] 1981	438 Large burns With INH	— 3.31 L/M² TBSA 5.37 L/M² TBSA	Same adults as in 1979 report Fluids given in the first 9 h are listed, expressed as liters/meter² TBSA
Scheulen & Munster,[6] 1982	48 INH 54 non-INH	14.5 L 9.7 L	Review of adults with burns of 10%–60% TBSA Inhalation injury exceeded calculated requirements by 37%
Navar et al,[7] 1985	51 INH 120 Non-INH	5.76 ± 0.39 3.98 ± 0.39	Review of children and adults with burns ≥25% TBSA INH subjects required more fluid and time to complete resuscitation
Herndon et al,[8] 1988	20 INH 14 non-INH	3.8 ± 1.5 2.3 ± 1.2	Adults with major burns LR alone used during the first 24 h
Darling et al,[9] 1996	100 INH	6.52 ± 0.26	All burn subjects with inhalation injuries Odds of death and ARDS increased progressively with fluids given
Dai et al,[10] 1998	26 INH 36 non-INH	3.1 ± 1.0 2.3 ± 0.8	Adults with burns ≥20% TBSA All subjects received colloid starting at 24 h
Engrav et al,[11] 2000	29/50 (58%)	5.2 ± 2.3	Multicenter review from 7 centers Requirements were greater in subjects with INH
Fluid creep in other situations			
Ivy et al,[2] 2000	98/109	9.36 (2.2–38.6)	Prospective evaluation of ACS, which developed in 2 subjects
Cartotto et al,[12] 2002	26/31 (84%)	6.7 ± 2.8	Retrospective evaluation of adults treated, 1998–2000 Most subjects exhibited fluid creep
Cancio et al,[13] 2004	56/89 (63%)	6.1 ± 0.2	Subjects resuscitated with the modified Brooke formula, 1987–1997
Friedrich et al,[14] 2004 Sullivan et al,[15] 2004	22 —	3.6 ± 1.1 (1970s) 8.0 ± 2.5 (2000)	Comparison of 11 patients resuscitated during 1975–79 with 11 patients matched for age, sex, and burn size, treated in 2000

(continued on next page)

Table 1
(continued)

Author, Year	Number of Subjects[a]	Resuscitation Received (mL/kg/% TBSA)[b]	Comments
Mitra et al,[16] 2006	49	5.58	Review of adults with burns ≥15% TBSA 73% required more than Parkland predictions but complications from fluid were minimal
Cochran et al,[17] 2007	101 —	9.4 ± 6.4 (albumin) 6.5 ± 4.4 (LR only)	Review of subjects who required albumin rescue for increasing fluid requirements compared with matched controls In multivariate analysis, use of albumin was associated with decreased mortality
Klein et al,[18] 2007	72	5.20	Multicenter review 56 subjects required ≤1.5 times Parkland estimates, 16 required more Inhalation injury not significant
Blumetti et al,[19] 2008	483	6.07	Review of adults with burns ≥19% TBSA Subjects were considered over-resuscitated whose urine output exceeded 1.0 mL/kg/h 210 subjects adequately resuscitated received 5.8 ± 2.3 mL/kg/% TBSA vs 6.1 ± 2.7 for over-resuscitated group
Dulhunty et al,[20] 2008	80	6.0 ± 2.3	Adults with burns ≥15% TBSA 36 subjects (45%) were poor responders and required more than 1/3 greater than Parkland Inhalation injury not significant
Chung et al,[21] 2009	58	3.8 ± 1.2 (Brooke) vs 5.9 ± 1.1 (Parkland)	Review of military burn transports Both Brooke and Parkland formulas were used Both resulted in infusion volumes in excess of predictions
Cartotto & Zhou,[22] 2010	196	6.3 ± 2.9	Review of adults with burns ≥15% TBSA 76% of subjects' fluids in excess of Parkland predictions No effect of INH Investigators noted a strong trend toward more frequent use of albumin

(continued on next page)

Author, Year	Number of Subjects[a]	Resuscitation Received (mL/kg/% TBSA)[b]	Comments
Table 1 *(continued)*			
Mason et al,[23] 2016	93/33	7.6	Multicenter review of adults Standard resuscitation was defined as 4–6 mL/kg/% TBSA 109 restricted subjects received less than this (2.9 mL/kg/%) 128 were within range (4.9 mL/kg/%), 93 exceeded it Restrictive subjects had higher risk of acute kidney injury

Abbreviations: ARDS, acute respiratory distress syndrome; TBSA, total body surface area; INH, inhalation injury.

[a] Subject numbers expressed as a fraction indicate the subjects within the reviewed cohort for whom excessive fluid requirements were reported.

[b] Unless otherwise stated, resuscitation listed consists of crystalloid fluids given in the first 24 hours following injury.

Data from Saffle JR. The phenomenon of "fluid creep" in acute burn resuscitation. J Burn Care Res 2007;28(3):382–95.

suggested that much more liberal opioid dosing might play a role, or even that the nature of burn injury had changed.

Regardless of the reasons, the reports in **Table 1** describe typical crystalloid requirements ranging from 4.6 to 9.4 mL/kg/% TBSA for patients with major burns, so that at least moderate fluid creep is a common and, to some extent, an expected finding. In acknowledgment of this, a very recent review of 330 adult patients from the influential Glue Grant consortium defined normal fluid resuscitation as 4 to 6 mL/kg/% TBSA and found that patients who resuscitated with abnormally low fluid requirements were at increased risk of acute kidney injury.[23]

Given its multiple causes and current emphasis on aggressive resuscitation, it is likely that some degree of fluid creep is here to stay, which prompts several questions: Is fluid creep really harmful? What constitutes over-resuscitation? What causes it? And, how could and/or should it be managed?

How Much Is Too Much?

The stated goal of burn resuscitation is simple: give as little fluid as possible while avoiding complications of under-resuscitation or over-resuscitation. Fluid formulas were initially developed to prevent early acute renal failure, which is now rare. Instead, serious complications of over-resuscitation are now a much bigger clinical problem. These complications include extremity compartment syndromes (including unburned extremities), massive swelling in the face and airway necessitating prolonged intubation, pleural effusions, and respiratory and cardiac failure.[20,28] ACS as a secondary consequence of fluid creep has become widely recognized as an uncommon but devastating clinical emergency with mortality of 75%.[2,29] Even more recently, elevated intraocular pressures leading to permanent blindness[30] has emerged as another horrific consequence linked to extreme over-resuscitation.

Clearly, there is such a thing as too much fluid but, in some situations, a certain amount of fluid creep may be appropriate. In Baxter's[5] experience, most patients with burns exceeding 70% TBSA died, many of resuscitation failure. Currently, patients with massive injuries commonly survive resuscitation well beyond Parkland confines. Baxter[5] noted that fluid requirements increase disproportionately with burn size and this has been confirmed repeatedly.[18,20] Cancio and colleagues[13] found requirements ranging from 4.0 mL/kg/% TBSA for moderate injuries to almost 6.0 mL/kg/% TBSA for burns of 80% to 100% TBSA. In this situation, fluid requirements may simply be a surrogate marker for burn severity and a necessary component of successful care.

In addition, the relationship between fluid volumes and edema-related complications is not straightforward. Some reports describe very low complication rates and mortality despite increased resuscitation volumes.[18,22] Patients have developed intra-abdominal hypertension and ACS after relatively normal resuscitation, whereas others tolerate extreme fluid volumes without difficulty. Total burn size, age, sepsis, and mechanical ventilation all correlate with development of ACS.[18] Markell and colleagues[31] reviewed 32 cases of ACS from among 1825 patients at Brooke Burn Center. They found that risk of ACS correlated closely with increasing burn size but not with indexed resuscitation volume. Risk of ACS and ocular hypertension increase most clearly only when fluids exceeded the Ivy index of 250 mL/kg, or a total (or predicted total) resuscitation volume of 6 mL/kg/% TBSA,[2,18] which should alert clinicians to institute corrective measures. Of interest is that these recent reports did not find that inhalation injury increased fluid requirements. Investigators postulated that endotracheal intubation, not inhalation injury itself, contributes to increased requirements. Also, the generous resuscitation given in many patients probably obscures the effects of inhalation injury.

Thus, although over-resuscitation can certainly be dangerous, aggressive resuscitation of patients with very large injuries, which was not practiced in Baxter's day, may not constitute over-resuscitation. This does not mean, however, that the goal of resuscitation has changed. Even patients with appropriate fluid creep may benefit from maneuvers to reduce fluid requirements.

Causes of Fluid Creep: Fluid Begets Fluid

The physiology of burn shock has been studied extensively.[32] (See review, in this issue.) During the first 8 to 12 hours following burn injury, capillary permeability in burned tissues is increased almost totally; fluid administered during this period ends up largely as edema. Leakage of even large protein molecules eliminates the oncotic pressure gradient necessary to maintain intravascular volume. In addition, this fluid leakage alters the densely configured collagen-hyaluronic interstitial matrix that ordinarily acts as a safety valve to edema formation. Instead, osmotically active fragments are produced that generate negative (sucking) interstitial pressure and enhanced compliance to continued fluid accumulation with little change in hydrostatic pressure. This persists even after capillary integrity is restored,[33] creating a cycle of ongoing capillary leakage and edema formation, which requires increasing volumes of crystalloid to satisfy.

This explains why fluid requirements that escalate mostly after the first 8 to 12 hours is a hallmark of fluid creep, and why excessive fluid given in the early postburn course predisposes to fluid creep later. Chung and colleagues[21] found that military burn patients started on the Parkland formula required 5.9 ± 1.1 mL/kg/% TBSA, compared with 3.8 ± 1.2 mL/kg/% TBSA for similar patients given the Brooke formula, despite identical targeted outcomes. They concluded that "a burn resuscitation that is begun at a higher fluid rate, results in more volume given during 24 hours."

Unfortunately, several trends in modern medicine favor excessive early crystalloid resuscitation and help explain why fluid creep has emerged at this point in time. First, overzealous resuscitation is common among well-intentioned emergency personnel who often overestimate burn size and follow trauma teachings to provide boluses or run intravenous lines wide open. As a result, patients frequently arrive at the burn center having received a major portion of their entire Parkland resuscitation within just a few hours.[12,16,20]

Second, burn clinicians have been influenced by goal-directed resuscitation in critical care, in which fluids are increased to normalize acidosis or achieve supranormal levels of cardiac output or oxygen utilization.[34] This approach initially seemed effective but, in subsequent analyses, has not proved superior to traditional treatment and clearly resulted in increased fluid volumes and ACS.[35] In burn patients, goal-directed resuscitation using as much as 4 times Parkland calculations has not improved survival and often failed to attain goal values.[36,37] This experience has confirmed earlier studies showing that cardiac output and other parameters require 18 to 24 hours to normalize following burn injury no matter what resuscitation is used. If invasive hemodynamic monitoring is of value at all, it is in selected high-risk patients, largely in avoiding errors in resuscitation.

Third, there is prejudice against colloid. As noted, colloid was eliminated from the 1979 consensus on burn resuscitation and other evidence that colloid was harmful encouraged practitioners to avoid its use.[38] In 1983, Goodwin and colleagues[39] found that a colloid-based regimen required less fluid than crystalloid resuscitation but led to progressive increases in lung water and higher mortality. This small study has influenced resuscitation practices for years, perhaps excessively so. More recent trials have shown no difference in outcomes with colloid use.[40,41] The alarming consequences of extreme fluid creep have stimulated many centers to reincorporate colloid into their resuscitation regimens, with success in limiting fluid requirements.

Clinicians not only turn fluids up in burn resuscitation, they are slow in turning them down. In several reports reviewed, average urine outputs exceeded 1 mL/kg/h, the upper limit usually mentioned for Parkland resuscitation. Cancio and colleagues[13] found that clinicians were less likely to reduce infusions in the face of increased urine output than they were to increase fluids for inadequate output. Blumetti and colleagues[19] found that patients who exceeded targeted urine outputs required more fluid (6.1 ± 2.7 mL/kg/% TBSA), although even patients resuscitated to appropriate urine outputs exhibited fluid creep (mean fluids 5.8 ± 2.3). This suggests that, although laxity in adherence to protocol contributes to fluid creep, its contribution may be relatively minor.

MANAGING FLUID CREEP

The presumed causes of fluid creep listed previously also indicate remedies that should halt or reverse progression of this problem. Strategies are given in the following sections.

Develop a Protocol

Successful resuscitation of major burn injuries requires the entire burn team. A clear protocol that everyone supports will help practitioners to restrict early fluid use, monitor and adjust changing requirements appropriately, and trigger aggressive strategies when predetermined alarm variables are reached. Because the causes of fluid creep described previously are multiple (and there well may be others), any resuscitation protocol must be flexible enough to deal with all of these issues as they present themselves.

Start Small

Fluid requirements immediately following burn injury are usually well below Parkland estimates and rise only later.[13] Other initial parameters, such as blood pressure, heart rate, and acid-base balance, are likely to reflect the injury itself more than resuscitation status. In the early postburn period, adjusting fluids to maintain urine output often means reducing fluid rates. Clinicians should be careful to restrict early fluids and encourage local emergency room personnel and emergency providers to avoid boluses and provide careful monitoring during transport. A host of computerized calculators and cell phone applications are available that have been shown to help inexperienced providers calculate burn size and fluid requirements more accurately, as well as aid burn professionals in adhering to protocol guidelines.[42–44]

Follow the Curve

Resuscitation requirements generally adhere fairly closely to Parkland predictions within the first 8 to 12 hours following burn injury and escalating resuscitation, even above predicted needs, may well be appropriate, particularly in patients with large injuries. However, fluid needs that continue to increase after this time are a hallmark of fluid creep and a signal to institute some strategy to reverse this trend. Calculating total administered fluids and predicting future needs will help make this decision. A prediction of 6 mL/kg/% TBSA or greater, or the Ivy index of 250 mL/kg, are ominous findings and should prompt corrective action.

Consider Colloid

In nearly every report of burn resuscitation the use of colloid has reduced total fluid requirements, limited edema in unburned tissues, and lessened or prevented extremity and ACSs.[30,45,46] However, routine colloid infusions early postburn when capillary permeability is high are unlikely to be helpful and many patients resuscitate uneventfully with crystalloids alone. For these reasons, colloid is probably best considered after 12 to 18 hours postinjury, either as a routine supplement or as rescue treatment of fluid creep. Some centers give a bolus of plasma at the end of 18 to 24 hours, as Baxter recommended.[19,47] Yowler and Fratianne[26] began albumin infusions beginning at 12 hours following burn injury when fluid requirements exceed 120% of predicted. Chung and colleagues[46] instituted colloid rescue when total fluid requirements were estimated to exceed 6 mL/kg/% TBSA.

Colloid use in burn resuscitation is now regaining popularity. More than half the centers responding in a recent international survey of resuscitation practices now incorporate colloid within the first 24 hours of injury.[48]

The University of Utah developed a strict resuscitation protocol in which 2.5% albumin in LR is added to resuscitation when hourly fluid requirements exceed twice the predicted values.[3] This has been almost invariably successful: starting albumin produces a dramatic increase in urine output and fluids can then be reduced rapidly.[49] Cochran and colleagues[17] found that albumin use was associated with decreased mortality in a multivariate logistic model.

Other Rescue Strategies

Several other resuscitation strategies can be helpful in reducing or halting fluid creep.

Hypertonic saline

Hypertonic saline solutions have been used in burn resuscitation for decades, require less fluid than isotonic crystalloid regimens, and can reduce the risk of ACS.[50,51]

However, significant hypernatremia and a possible risk of acute kidney injury complicate this therapy, so careful monitoring is essential.

High-dose ascorbic acid
High-dose ascorbic acid (vitamin C) infusions in conjunction with standard crystalloid
resuscitation have been shown to reduce total fluid requirements in severe burns.[52]
Though some concern exists over a possible increase in the incidence of acute renal
failure, this method is attractive because it can be started preemptively, without waiting for the development of worrisome fluid creep. Use of this modality is also gaining in
popularity.

As a last resort or emergency treatment, plasmapheresis has been shown to arrest
fluid creep, and may directly reduce abdominal hypertension.[53] The procedure is invasive and expensive; it should be considered only rarely if other measures are used
proactively.

SUMMARY

In the years since Pruitt defined fluid creep, a variety of strategies to prevent or reduce
the complications of excessive fluid resuscitation have been incorporated into more
responsive resuscitation regimens. Several of these are now recognized in updated
guidelines for fluid therapy.[54] Has the burn care community succeeded in pushing
the pendulum back? Pruitt[55] himself seems to think so, commenting recently that,
"Fluid resuscitation has moved from inadequate to excessive and is now returning
to adequate." With appropriate attention to detail, fluid creep can be successfully
managed in almost all patients, even while normal resuscitation has been redefined.
In the future, successful resuscitation will likely become more flexible still, perhaps
consisting of a menu of protocols for different injuries, using computerized decision
support to monitor the essential details of patient response, and producing instanta-
neous adjustments in fluid management.

REFERENCES

1. Pruitt BA Jr. Protection from excessive resuscitation: "pushing the pendulum
   back". J Trauma 2000;49(3):567–8.
2. Ivy ME, Atweh NA, Palmer J, et al. Intra-abdominal hypertension and abdominal
   compartment syndrome in burn patients. J Trauma 2000;49(3):387–91.
3. Saffle JR. The phenomenon of "fluid creep" in acute burn resuscitation. J Burn
   Care Res 2007;28(3):382–95.
4. Baxter CR. Problems and complications of burn shock resuscitation. Surg Clin
   North Am 1978;58(6):1313–22.
5. Baxter CR. Guidelines for fluid resuscitation. J Trauma 1981;21:687–92.
6. Scheulen JJ, Munster AM. The Parkland formula in patients with burns and inhalation injury. J Trauma 1982;22(10):869–71.
7. Navar PD, Saffle JR, Warden GD. Effect of inhalation injury on fluid resuscitation
   requirements after thermal injury. Am J Surg 1985;150(6):716–20.
8. Herndon DN, Barrow RE, Linares HA, et al. Inhalation injury in burned patients:
   effects and treatment. Burns Incl Therm Inj 1988;14(5):349–56.
9. Darling GE, Keresteci MA, Ibanez D, et al. Pulmonary complications in inhalation
   injuries with associated cutaneous burn. J Trauma 1996;40(1):83–9.
10. Dai NT, Chen TM, Cheng TY, et al. The comparison of early fluid therapy in exten-
    sive flame burns between inhalation and noninhalation injuries. Burns 1998;24(7):
    671–5.

11. Engrav LH, Colescott PL, Kemalyan N, et al. A biopsy of the use of the Baxter formula to resuscitate burns or do we do it like Charlie did it? J Burn Care Rehabil 2000;21(2):91–5.

12. Cartotto RC, Innes M, Musgrave MA, et al. How well does the Parkland formula estimate actual fluid resuscitation volumes? J Burn Care Rehabil 2002;23(4): 258–65.

13. Cancio LC, Chavez S, Alvarado-Ortega M, et al. Predicting increased fluid requirements during the resuscitation of thermally injured patients. J Trauma 2004;56(2):404–13 [discussion: 13–4].

14. Friedrich JB, Sullivan SR, Engrav LH, et al. Is supra-Baxter resuscitation in burn patients a new phenomenon? Burns 2004;30(5):464–6.

15. Sullivan SR, Friedrich JB, Engrav LH, et al. "Opioid creep" is real and may be the cause of "fluid creep". Burns 2004;30(6):583–90.

16. Mitra B, Fitzgerald M, Cameron P, et al. Fluid resuscitation in major burns. ANZ J Surg 2006;76(1–2):35–8.

17. Cochran A, Morris SE, Edelman LS, et al. Burn patient characteristics and outcomes following resuscitation with albumin. Burns 2007;33(1):25–30.

18. Klein MB, Hayden D, Elson C, et al. The association between fluid administration and outcome following major burn: a multicenter study. Ann Surg 2007;245(4): 622–8.

19. Blumetti J, Hunt JL, Arnoldo BD, et al. The Parkland formula under fire: is the criticism justified? J Burn Care Res 2008;29(1):180–6.

20. Dulhunty JM, Boots RJ, Rudd MJ, et al. Increased fluid resuscitation can lead to adverse outcomes in major-burn injured patients, but low mortality is achievable. Burns 2008;34(8):1090.

21. Chung KK, Wolf SE, Cancio LC, et al. Resuscitation of severely burned military casualties: fluid begets more fluid. J Trauma 2009;67(2):231.

22. Cartotto R, Zhou A. Fluid creep: the pendulum hasn't swung back yet. J Burn Care Res 2010;31(4):551–8.

23. Mason SA, Nathens AB, Finnerty CC, et al. Hold the pendulum: rates of acute kidney injury are increased in patients who receive resuscitation volumes less than predicted by the Parkland Equations. Ann Surg 2016. [Epub ahead of print].

24. Moncrief JA. Effect of various fluid regimens and pharmacologic agents on the circulatory hemodynamics of the immediate postburn period. Ann Surg 1966; 164(4):723–52.

25. Schwartz SI. Supportive therapy in burn care. Consensus summary on fluid resuscitation. J Trauma 1979;19(11 Suppl):876–7.

26. Yowler CJ, Fratianne RB. Current status of burn resuscitation. Clin Plast Surg 2000;27(1):1–10.

27. Hughes KR, Armstrong RF, Brough MD, et al. Fluid requirements of patients with burns and inhalation injuries in an intensive care unit. Intensive Care Med 1989; 15(7):464–6.

28. Zak AL, Harrington DT, Barillo DJ, et al. Acute respiratory failure that complicates the resuscitation of pediatric patients with scald injuries. J Burn Care Rehabil 1999;20(5):391–9.

29. Strang SG, Van Lieshout EM, Breedervelt RS, et al. A systematic review of intra-abdominal pressure in severely burned patients. Burns 2014;40(1):9–16.

30. Medina MA 3rd, Moore DA, Cairns BA. A case series: bilateral ischemic optic neuropathy secondary to large volume fluid resuscitation in critically ill burn patients. Burns 2015;41(3):e19–23.

31. Markell KW, Renz EM, White CE, et al. Abdominal complications after severe burns. J Am Coll Surg 2009;208(5):940–9.
32. Demling RH. The burn edema process: current concepts. J Burn Care Rehabil 2005;26(3):207–27.
33. Leape LL. Initial changes in burns: tissue changes in burned and unburned skin of rhesus monkeys. J Trauma 1970;10(6):488–92.
34. Fleming A, Bishop M, Shoemaker W, et al. Prospective trial of supranormal values as goals of resuscitation in severe trauma. Arch Surg 1992;127(10):1175–9 [discussion: 1179–81].
35. Balogh Z, McKinley BA, Cocanour CS, et al. Supranormal trauma resuscitation causes more cases of abdominal compartment syndrome. Arch Surg 2003; 138(6):637–42 [discussion: 42–3].
36. Barton RG, Saffle JR, Morris SE, et al. Resuscitation of thermally injured patients with oxygen transport criteria as goals of therapy. J Burn Care Rehabil 1997;18(1 Pt 1):1–9.
37. Holm C, Mayr M, Tegeler J, et al. A clinical randomized study on the effects of invasive monitoring on burn shock resuscitation. Burns 2004;30(8):798–807.
38. Alderson P, Bunn F, Lefebvre C, et al. Human albumin solution for resuscitation and volume expansion in critically ill patients. Cochrane Database Syst Rev 2002;(1):CD001208.
39. Goodwin CW, Dorethy J, Lam V, et al. Randomized trial of efficacy of crystalloid and colloid resuscitation on hemodynamic response and lung water following thermal injury. Ann Surg 1983;197(5):520–31.
40. Finfer S, Bellomo R, Boyce N, et al. A comparison of albumin and saline for fluid resuscitation in the intensive care unit. N Engl J Med 2004;350(22):2247–56.
41. Cooper AB, Cohn SM, Zhang HS, et al. Five percent albumin for adult burn shock resuscitation: lack of effect on daily multiple organ dysfunction score. Transfusion 2006;46(1):80–9.
42. Neuwalder JM, Sampson C, Breuing KH, et al. A review of computer-aided body surface area determination: SAGE II and EPRI's 3D Burn Vision. J Burn Care Rehabil 2002;23(1):55–9 [discussion: 54].
43. Kamolz LP, Lumenta DB, Parvizi D, et al. Smartphones and burn size estimation: "Rapid Burn Assessor". Ann Burns Fire Disasters 2014;27(2):101–4.
44. Salinas J, Chung KK, Mann EA, et al. Computerized decision support system improves fluid resuscitation following severe burns: an original study. Crit Care Med 2011;39(9):2031–8.
45. Cartotto R, Callum J. Review of the use of human albumin in burn patients. J Burn Care Res 2012;33(6):702–17.
46. Chung KK, Blackbourne LH, Wolf SE, et al. Evolution of burn resuscitation in operation Iraqi freedom. J Burn Care Res 2006;27(5):606–11.
47. Warden G. Fluid resuscitation and early management. In: Herndon D, editor. Total burn care. Philadelphia: WB Saunders; 2007. p. 107–18.
48. Greenhalgh DG. Burn resuscitation: the results of the ISBI/ABA survey. Burns 2010;36(2):176–82.
49. Lawrence A, Faraklas I, Watkins H, et al. Colloid administration normalizes resuscitation ratio and ameliorates "fluid creep". J Burn Care Res 2010;31(1):40–7.
50. Monafo WW. The treatment of burn shock by the intravenous and oral administration of hypertonic lactated saline solution. J Trauma 1970;10(7):575–86.
51. Oda J, Ueyama M, Yamashita K, et al. Hypertonic lactated saline resuscitation reduces the risk of abdominal compartment syndrome in severely burned patients. J Trauma 2006;60(1):64–71.

52. Kahn SA, Beers RJ, Lentz CS. Resuscitation after severe burn injury using high-dose ascorbic acid: a retrospective review. J Burn Care Res 2011;32(1):110–7.

53. Mosier MM, DeChristopher PJ, Gamelli RL. Use of therapeutic plasma exchange in the burn unit: a review of the literature. J Burn Care Res 2013;34(3):289–98.

54. Pham TN, Cancio LC, Gibran NS. American Burn Association practice guidelines: burn shock resuscitation. J Burn Care Res 2008;29(1):257–66.

55. Pruitt BA. Reflection: evolution of the field over seven decades. Surg Clin North Am 2014;94(4):721–40.

Protocolized Resuscitation of Burn Patients

Leopoldo C. Cancio, MD[a],*, Jose Salinas, PhD[a], George C. Kramer, PhD[b]

KEYWORDS

- Fluid resuscitation • Burns • Decision making—Computer-Assisted
- Decision support systems - Clinical

KEY POINTS

- Fluid resuscitation of patients with burn shock requires careful hourly titration (up or down) of fluid infusion rates. Over-resuscitation has become more common (fluid creep).
- Patients who receive greater than 250 mL/kg during the first 24 hours following burn injury are at risk of abdominal compartment syndrome (ACS) and other complications. ACS in burn patients is highly lethal despite decompressive laparotomy.
- Paper-based flow sheets and clinical practice guidelines for burn resuscitation are associated with improved outcomes.
- Computerized decision support tools have been developed to assist providers during the resuscitation process.

INTRODUCTION

The concept of formulas, algorithms, and protocols for the fluid resuscitation of severely injured burn patients is not new, but recent advances in information technology have enabled development of computerized versions of these methods. This article reviews these techniques and proposes a framework for evaluating them.

An understanding of the pathophysiology of burn shock as involving the loss of plasma-like fluid from the intravascular space into the interstitium led to the use of

---

Disclosures: The opinions or assertions contained herein are the private views of the authors and are not to be construed as official or as reflecting the official views of the Department of the Army or the Department of Defense.

Funding Sources: Funded by the Combat Casualty Care Research Program of the US Army Medical Research and Materiel Command, Fort Detrick, MD.

Conflicts of Interest: L.C. Cancio and J. Salinas are coinventors of Burn Resuscitation Decision Support System (BRDSS), which has been licensed by the US Army to Arcos, Inc. They have assigned their rights to the US Army, but would receive a small portion of any royalties. G.C. Kramer is a coinventor of BRDSS and is a principal member of Arcos, Inc.

[a] US Army Institute of Surgical Research, 3698 Chambers Pass, JBSA Fort Sam Houston, TX 78234-6315, USA; [b] Department of Anesthesiology, University of Texas Medical Branch at Galveston, Galveston, TX 77555-1102, USA

* Corresponding author.

E-mail address: leopoldo.c.cancio.civ@mail.mil

plasma for fluid resuscitation.[1] Following the Cocoanut Grove fire of 1942, fluid resuscitation formulas were proposed and widely adopted that used varying concentrations of plasma and crystalloid solutions during the first 24 to 48 hours following burn injury.[2] There was a gradual movement away from plasma over the ensuing years.[3] This reflected the observation that hypovolemic shock causes an extracellular fluid deficit,[4] and created a focus on correcting this deficit with crystalloid solutions.[5] During the 1960s, researchers at the Brooke and Parkland hospitals in Texas developed formulas which used only lactated Ringer's (LR) solution, and no plasma, for the first 24 hours following burn injury.[5,6] The modified Brooke formula (which estimates the first 24-hour volume as LR solution, 2 mL/kg/total body surface area burned [TBSA], with half of this delivered over the first 8 hours) and the Parkland formula (similar to Brooke but 4 mL/kg/TBSA) are the most commonly used formulas for resuscitation of adult burn patients today.[7] Albumin replaced plasma in most resuscitation regimens and was used primarily during the second 24 hours, at a dose of 0.3 to 0.5 mL/kg/TBSA for the day.[8] Subsequently, the utility of colloid solutions before the 24th hour in selected patients reemerged (early albumin), especially in those in whom early resuscitation performance indicated a risk of large-volume resuscitation.[9–11]

Formulas for the resuscitation of burn patients are widely accepted. However, slavish adherence to a formula without adjustment of the fluid infusion rate based on physiologic response is to be condemned. A burn resuscitation formula provides a starting point; the patient's care is then tailored in response to therapy. This can be viewed as a basic example of personalized medicine.[12] For many patients, the volumes infused are greater than those predicted by the formula, be it the Parkland, Brooke, or some other formula.[13,14]

In the absence of any randomized controlled trials of burn resuscitation formulas, a retrospective study was performed by Chung and colleagues[15] in combat casualties, some of whom were started at 2, and some at 4 mL/kg/TBSA. This study showed that fluid begets more fluid: if one starts resuscitation at the rate predicted by the 2 mL/kg/TBSA formula, then the actual infusion volume approximates 4 mL/kg/TBSA by the end of the 24-hour period. If one starts at the rate predicted by the 4 mL/kg/TBSA formula, then the actual infusion volume approximates 6 mL/kg/TBSA. A possible explanation for this is that the microvasculature is more sensitive to hydrostatic pressure gradients during the initial hours following burn injury. In other words, extra fluid infused under a high-volume strategy during the early hours following burn injury is simply lost.[16] Another explanation is that excessive crystalloid therapy damages the glycocalyx, which is known to maintain normal capillary permeability.[17] Furthermore, burn resuscitation with LR solution has been shown to wash components of the glycocalyx out of the microcirculation.[18]

How exactly to adjust the fluid infusion rate based on physiologic response has constituted the art of fluid resuscitation. The main indicator of the adequacy of resuscitation in burn patients remains the hourly urine output (UO).[19] The reasons for using hourly UO are that it is easily measured (once a Foley catheter has been placed), it reflects glomerular filtration rate and renal blood flow, and it is a surrogate for end organ perfusion and an indirect correlate of cardiac output. The target range for UO in burn resuscitation is 30 to 50 mL per hour in adults, or 0.5 to 1.0 mL/kg/h. Recently, some burn experts have argued for a lower target of 0.25 to 0.5 mL/kg/h, in an attempt to counter the trend toward over-resuscitation (R. Sheridan, MD, personal communication, 2016). Changes in infusion rate are made about once an hour. This means that the fluid infusion rate should be increased if the UO is less than the target, and decreased if the UO is greater than the target. In practice, the recent literature suggests that clinicians are more likely to increase the infusion rate than they are to decrease it, and more likely to accept a high UO than a low one.[14,20] That is, they err on the side of over-resuscitation rather than on the side of under-resuscitation.

Whatever the cause, the effects of over-resuscitation in patients with burn shock can be severe. Ivy and colleagues[21] identified the infusion of 250 mL/kg during the first 24 hours following burn injury as increasing the risk of abdominal compartment syndrome (ACS). ACS in burn patients is associated with greatly increased mortality. This is particularly true if ACS requires treatment with a decompressive laparotomy. In the context of edematous tissues and abdominal contents, abdominal domain is easily lost, and the physiologic stress of an open abdomen in combination with extensive body burns is rarely survivable. Other complications of fluid overload in burn patients include: (1) extremity compartment syndrome,[22,23] (2) pulmonary and laryngeal edema,[24] and (3) malperfusion of burn wounds (leading to conversion of partial thickness to full thickness wounds, and to decreased success of skin grafting procedures). This concatenation of complications led Pruitt[25] to describe the phenomenon of fluid creep, and to insist on the need for greater discipline in the execution of burn shock resuscitation.

PROTOCOLIZED BURN RESUSCITATION

The problem, in brief, is how to achieve not just personalized medicine, but precision medicine, during the titration of infusion rates during resuscitation. Tighter and optimal control of fluid resuscitation is needed. Although much of this article focuses on computerized burn resuscitation, there is value in a rigorous paper-based approach. Faced with a high rate of ACS in burned combat casualties from the recent wars in Iraq and Afghanistan, Ennis and colleagues,[10] at the US Army Burn Center, promulgated a paper-based burn resuscitation flow sheet and set of clinical practice guidelines. Implementation of these guidelines was assiduously carried out across the military health care system via the newly organized Joint Theater Trauma System (JTTS). Modeled after civilian trauma systems, the JTTS provided a mechanism for rapid performance improvement that included, for example, weekly teleconferences in which the care of seriously wounded US personnel was critiqued.[26] The paper flow sheet provided a mechanism for better documentation and for achieving continuity in situational awareness during the numerous hand-offs that characterize patient flow through the aeromedical evacuation system. It should be noted that the JTTS burn resuscitation flow sheet did not provide for hourly specific recommendations based on the patient's UO. However, in burned combat casualties greater than 30% TBSA, Ennis and colleagues[10] found that guideline implementation decreased ACS from 16% to 5% ($P = .06$), mortality from 31% to 18% ($P = .11$), and the composite endpoint of ACS and mortality from 36% to 18% ($P = .03$).

A widely recognized nurse-driven protocol for fluid resuscitation was developed at the University of Utah. It provides for hourly adjustment of infusion rates based on UO, and timely rescue with albumin of patients on course for a large-volume resuscitation. Indications for initiation of albumin included (1) edema-related complications or (2) infusion of twice the Parkland formula prediction for 2 or more consecutive hours. Albumin was initiated at one-third the hourly LR solution rate at the time of the change, and the LR rate was decreased to two-thirds of the previous LR solution rate. In children, this strategy rapidly restored the hourly input-to-output ratio to that of crystalloid-only patients.[27] These investigators evaluated their experience with the protocol to determine whether large-volume resuscitation was the result of error by nurses. They found that 48% of patients were resuscitated with crystalloid alone, with the remainder receiving crystalloid and albumin. The crystalloid-only group received 4.7 mL/kg/TBSA, and the albumin-rescue group received 7.5 mL/kg/TBSA. Nursing adherence to the written protocol was impeccable, with 1% error between predicted and actual fluid infusion rates. The investigators speculated that even earlier institution of albumin in those patients whose baseline characteristics predict eventual albumin rescue might help further reduce the infused volumes in that group.[28]

COMPUTERIZED BURN RESUSCITATION

Because fluid resuscitation is mainly a question of adjusting the infusion rate based on the UO, a negative-feedback-controlled system, similar to a thermostat, can be envisioned. However, a thermostat is a simple, on-off device, and a similar approach in a burn patient would subject him or her to repeated cycles of ischemia, reperfusion, and volume overload.[29] More sophisticated control systems are required in this patient population, and may incorporate simple controller lookup tables or more complicated techniques such as proportional-integral-derivative (PID), fuzzy-logic, or model-based control.

A PID controller takes into account 3 inputs describing the difference between the patient's actual state and the desired state: proportional, integral, and derivative.[30] Proportional refers to the magnitude of this difference. Integral refers to the area under curve for the difference over a defined period of time. Derivative refers to the rate of change of the difference over a period of time. For example, if a patient's UO output is 20, 15, and 10 mL per hour over the last 3 hours, and the desired UO is 40 mL per hour, then the proportional term is 40 to 10 = 30 mL/h, the integral term over 3 hours is (40–20) + (40–15) + (40–10) = 20 + 25 + 30 = 75 mL/h, and the derivative term over 3 hours is (10–20)/(3–1) = −5 mL/h. Each of these values is then individually multiplied by a coefficient that provides the appropriate changes to the infusion rate to achieve the desired UO. The initial weight given the individual coefficients in the PID control equation can be determined using a variety of manual and/or automated approaches; however, they may need to be modified (tuned) based on controller performance. Thirty-five years ago, PID control was used to perform closed-loop resuscitation in a canine burn model by Bowman and Westenskow[31] at the University of Utah. PID control was used more recently by Hoskins and colleagues[30] to perform closed-loop resuscitation of sheep with 40% TBSA burns. The controller performed as well as a human technician using a look-up table with respect to UO, infusion rates, and infusion volumes. The closed-loop group demonstrated lower hourly variation in UO and infusion rate, and less frequent hours in which UO was less than the target.

Fuzzy-logic control is an extension of fuzzy theory, which was developed by Dr Lotfi Zadeh[32] to explain concepts that cannot be defined by an exact value, and situations in which a degree of uncertainty or vagueness exists. Such scenarios are particularly common in medicine. For example, one clinician may define hypotension as mean arterial pressure (MAP) less than 60 mm Hg, whereas another may consider hypotension as MAP <55 mm Hg. Similarly, clinicians may have different definitions for normal and high blood pressures. Combining all definitions will create a distribution that defines blood pressure. A similar approach can be applied to definitions of hypovolemia. Drawing clear distinctions between these states may be difficult and there may be overlap. In many cases, overlap of fuzzy sets will lead to definitions that have partial membership in multiple sets (ie, a small percentage of the hypotension distribution may overlap with the distribution of normotension). In contrast, classic or Boolean logic permits only "yes" or "no" membership in a set. By providing a mathematical framework for transforming values to or from fuzzy distributions, a fuzzy control system can be implemented to handle biological situations that are not well defined.

Fuzzy-logic control has been used in several critical care applications[33] and to include resuscitation of hemorrhagic shock to a target blood pressure in sheep by Ying and colleagues.[34]

Model-based controllers incorporate a knowledge base concerning a patient's physiology and/or pathophysiology. This knowledge base is then used to determine appropriate values for the infusion rate based on what the controller knows about the patient (ie, the physiology embedded in the software). For example, if the user requires the patient to have a 40 mL per hour output for the next hour, the controller can determine what the correct infusion rate should be based on its vascular model. One of the advantages of model-based controllers is that, depending on the accuracy of the model, the system may not require feedback input.

There are several approaches for model implementation in model-based controllers. Early approaches incorporated strict mathematical representations for known physiologic responses (ie, implementation of Guyton's models). These approaches have the advantage of being well understood; however, computational requirements for implementing such complex models may not be feasible in many cases. Other types of common model representations include compartment-based approaches (in which the model is limited to physiologic responses from a limited number of organ systems) or statistical models (which use probabilistic distributions to represent a patient's physiology). More complex approaches may include use of machine-learning models, and hybrid systems, which combine several types of approaches to get both accurate and computationally efficient results. One of the main disadvantages of model-based systems is the lack of a thorough understanding of a patient's pathophysiology. When developing models for the critical-care environment, how to incorporate an individual patient's responses to the injury and/or procedures is the subject of ongoing research.

Hedlund and colleagues[35] described a computerized simulation of human physiology intended to model burn or trauma patients. The model calculated 150 variables and contained 6 modules (systemic circulation; microcirculation; endocrine system; renal system; electrolyte, urea, and protein distribution; and water distribution). One of the points made by the investigators is that the model can be used for in silico trialing of fluid resuscitation regimens before their implementation in humans.[36] Roa and colleagues[37] built a model of the response to burn injury that included the interactions between the intracellular and extracellular compartments, capillary dynamics in burned and unburned tissue, systemic hemodynamics, lymphatics in burned and unburned tissue, and renal function.[38] This model was used to develop, and to evaluate in silico, a fluid resuscitation protocol that was then implemented in human burn patients. However, the computer did not guide or perform the new resuscitation procedure.[39] Ampratwum and colleagues[40] developed a 3-compartment model of the microcirculation: the blood, the injured interstitium, and the uninjured interstitium. In this model, fluid and albumin is exchanged between these compartments and the equations describing the Starling forces between the compartments change over time following burn injury. The investigators point out the challenge involved in estimating values for certain physiologic parameters that are difficult or impossible to measure directly. These efforts indicate the potential for modeling human physiology following burn injury but, to date, implementation at the bedside of a model-based controller has not, to the authors' knowledge, been achieved.

Control systems can also be classified according to how much control the system exerts over the process versus how much control is exerted by the human provider. The authors define the following 7 levels of automation: (1) enhanced data display, (2) predictive support, (3) decision support, (4) open-loop control, (5) closed-loop control with human over-ride, (6) fully autonomous closed-loop control, and (7) hybrid open-loop and closed-loop-control systems. Each level incorporates increasing levels of implementation complexity (with associated increases in risk). Enhanced data display provides the user with better graphical displays, for example, by bringing together data, which, though clinically or physiologically interconnected, are housed in disparate locations. Furthermore, it provides user-friendly data visualization and enhanced provider situational awareness. For example, the UO and fluid infusion data may not be visible on the same page in the electronic medical record (EMR), even though these are the basic data elements needed to intelligently perform burn shock resuscitation. An example of this is shown in **Fig. 1**. Predictive support generates a prediction of the near-term future for a patient based on her or his performance during the recent past (including knowledge of the patient characteristics, if available). This can be done using a graphical display designed to facilitate the user's own prediction. It can be done based on an empirically developed statistical model, a support vector machine, Bayesian prediction, or an artificial neural network. An example is provided in **Fig. 2**. Knowledge that a patient is on course for a bad outcome, such as over-resuscitation, enables the user to consider altering course, for example, by changing the rate or type of fluids infused. Decision support adds a recommendation to the prediction. In the case of burn resuscitation, a decision support system may provide an hourly recommendation for a change in the fluid infusion rate (**Fig. 3**). Such recommendations require an internal logic, set of rules, or algorithm.

Open-loop control envisions a feedback loop as shown in **Fig. 4**. The components of this loop include the patient, a set of sensors (eg, a single digital urimeter), a computer, and a set of effectors (eg, one or more fluid infusion pumps). In the case of open-loop control, the computer receives the hourly UO data from the patient and calculates a new infusion rate. A human provider must approve and choose to implement this infusion rate, for example, by clicking on a menu item. The computer then carries out the infusion rate change by sending an instruction to the fluid infusion pump. Thus, the human is always in the loop and is also able to change the recommendation of the computer if desired. Closed-loop control envisions the same feedback loop, except that human approval is not necessary for the system to function. Closed-loop control with human override allows the provider to step in and modify care if desired. Fully autonomous closed-loop control is a state in which no human intervention occurs during normal operation. A hybrid system would include closed-loop control for much of

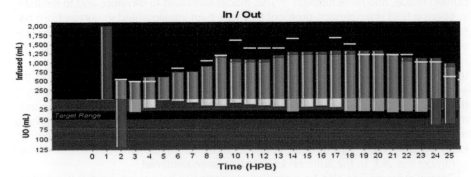

Fig. 1. Enhanced data display. Screen shot from Burn Resuscitation Decision Support System (BRDSS), showing simultaneous display of the fluid infusion rate and the UO rate for each hour postburn. Preburn-unit (eg, prehospital and referring hospital) fluids are shown on the left.

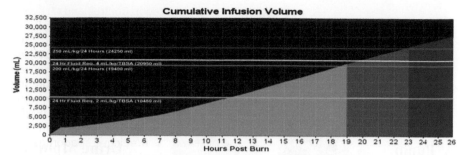

Fig. 2. Predictive support. Screen shot from BRDSS, showing cumulative infusion volume. The area under the curve changes color from green, to orange, to red, as the patient reaches 200 mL/kg and then 250 mL/kg during the first 24 hours postburn. Lines are drawn horizontally to indicate the 200 mL/kg, 250 mL/kg, 2 mL/kg/TBSA, and 4 mL/kg/TBSA thresholds.

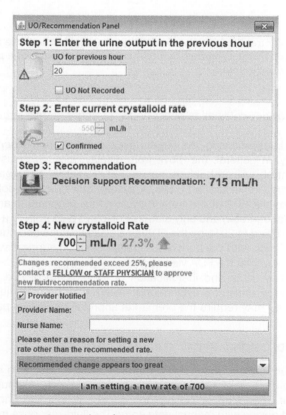

Fig. 3. Decision support. Screen shot from BRDSS, showing interactive window used by bedside nurse at the top of each postburn hour. The current fluid infusion rate and the recommended new rate are displayed. The nurse is free to either comply with or to modify the recommendation. Note also that in this case, communication with a physician is prompted because of a greater than 25% change in the recommended fluid infusion rate.

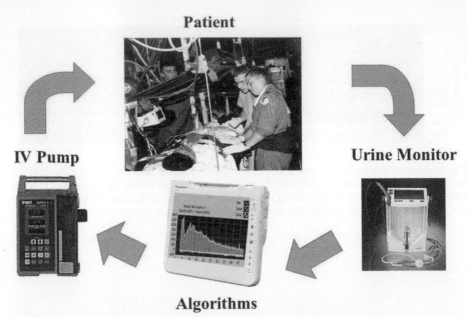

Fig. 4. Open-loop control. In this embodiment, the provider must approve an action, which is then implemented by the computer. In a fully closed-loop scenario, the provider is taken out of the loop. IV, intravenous.

the time, with provider notification either hourly or under certain circumstances (eg, hypotension).

The regulatory implications for the various levels of automation described previously vary substantially. In general, the move from display, through decision support, to autonomous control, will probably bring greater regulatory requirements from the US Food and Drug Administration (FDA). A system that functions solely as an EMR is not regulated by the FDA at this time. A system that connects to a medical device (eg, a pump and/or urimeter) and only stores or displays data is likely a medical device data system, classified in 2011 by the FDA as a class I device and subject to general controls.[41] Experience with the burn resuscitation decision support system (see later discussion) indicated that the FDA viewed this as a class II medical device, subject to the 510K regulatory route and identification of a predicate device. Depending on perceived risk to the patient, a closed-loop system may be classified as a class III medical device and may require the premarket approval regulatory pathway.

COMPUTERIZED DECISION SUPPORT: CLINICAL EXPERIENCE

The US Army Burn Center developed a burn resuscitation decision support system (BRDSS) to help guide fluid resuscitation during burn shock. Although theoretically capable of either open-loop or closed-loop control, it was first implemented as a decision-support device with manual data entry. The fluid-response model embodied in the software includes the following concepts. First, a retrospective review of data from patients resuscitated without BRDSS was performed. The fluid infusion rate and the UO for each hour postburn for this derivation data set were recorded. The nonlinear relationship between fluid input and UO was determined as a function of the postburn hour. Thus, for a given postburn hour, the amount of fluid required to produce a change in UO can be estimated. Second, these predictions were modified by consideration of the patient's TBSA and weight, such that a higher burn size and a higher weight generate more aggressive infusion rate recommendations. Third, linear regression of the last 3 hours' UO is performed. This is used to predict the next hour's UO. A recommendation is then generated for the next hour's infusion rate to keep the UO within target. Finally, as the UO approaches the target, the recommendation is dampened to reduce overshoot.[42]

This program was introduced at the Burn Center as a performance improvement project. Critical to the implementation process was a weekly multidisciplinary decision support team meeting. The purpose of this meeting was to review both user experience with the system, and system performance, over the previous week. Thus, experience with actual patients was used to optimize the system. Among the improvements that resulted from this spiral development process were the addition (and subsequent modification) of business rules. These rules were empirically derived from real world experience with the system and with patients. Examples of such rules include the following: (1) Do not recommend more than 2000 mL per hour. (2) Do not recommend a sustained rate of more than 1500 mL per hour. (3) Alert the provider if the patient has received more than 250 mL/kg (before the 24th hour), the Ivy Index predicting increased risk of ACS. (4) Alert the provider if the patient has received more than 200 mL/kg and is thus en route to exceeding the Ivy Index. (5) Prompt the user not to decrease the fluid infusion rate if the patient is hypotensive. (6) Do not decrease the infusion rate by more than 40% each hour. (7) Do not decrease the infusion rate below the maintenance rate of 125 mL per hour. (8) Prompt the user to obtain certain laboratory values, such as base deficit and lactate, every 6 hours. (9) Many of the above alerts encourage communication between the bedside nurse and the attending physician. It is likely that different burn centers may want to modify these business rules according to local practice.

This last point is, the authors believe, a key advantage of a program like this. The program identifies key events (eg, patient deterioration) and prompts communication. Thus, rather than remove the physician from the process, the system is intended to increase the situational awareness of the team at these critical time points, and to generate a shared vocabulary or mental model between nurse and physician about the nature of the problem to be solved. These events should be distinguished from typical alarms in an intensive care unit (ICU), such as blood pressure alarms on a vital signs monitor, in that the former contain contextual information. For example, the program identifies hypotension in the context of a brisk UO prediction, and a conversation between nurse and physician is suggested to balance these 2 apparently disparate findings. The authors emphasize that these concepts did not appear ex vacuo in the development of this program but could only be elucidated during group discussion and review of many patient resuscitation experiences.

This work led to development of a commercial product, Burn Navigator (Arcos, Inc, Houston, TX, USA), which is currently implemented on a rugged laptop computer. It was classified as a class II medical device by the FDA and approved under the 510K pathway. During device evaluation, the FDA required videotaped human-factors testing using simulated patients and both experienced and inexperienced bedside providers. This work was conducted under the supervision of an experienced burn ICU nurse at the US Army Burn Center and led to several practical and useful improvements in the device. The authors emphasize the utility of this type of evaluation for a system intended for use in clinical care of patients. It is noteworthy that similar testing is not required during the development of EMRs.[43]

Table 1 Findings from burn resuscitation decision support system experience		
Year	Author	Findings
2006	Salinas	UO was frequently above target during resuscitation. Only 40% of instances of out-of-range UO resulted in appropriate change in IR.
2010	Salinas	Following rapid increase, maximum IR occurred on average at 9 h postburn, followed by a gradual decline.
2011	Salinas	83% of DS recommendations were accepted. Providers more likely to follow DS recommendations after first 8 h postburn.
2012	Salinas	A decrease in IR occurred on average 3 h after initiation of albumin, especially with early use during hours 8–16 postburn.
2012	Kramer	Severe oliguria (<0.2 mL/kg/h) was more common in nonsurvivors than survivors.
2013	Salinas	Patients with inhalation injury received 4.2 mL/kg/TBSA, vs those without received 2.9 mL/kg/TBSA.
2013	Kramer	Nonresponder hours (low UO despite high IR) were more common in nonsurvivors.
2013	Serio	Female subjects received more fluid than male subjects (4.79 mL/kg/TBSA vs 3.44 mL/kg/TBSA).
2014	Salinas	FT burn size was an independent predictor of FR volume: 2.2 mL/kg for each percent increase in FT size.
2014	Salinas	Grade III-IV IAH was seen in 13% of subjects, and required infusion of a volume of ≥280 mL/kg during the first 24 h postburn.

All studies except the first were performed after the introduction of BRDSS for decision support in the US Army Burn Center. The first study was performed to support BRDSS algorithm development.

Abbreviations: DS, decision support; FR, fluid resuscitation; FT, full thickness; IAH, intra-abdominal hypertension; IR, infusion rate.

Data from Proceedings of the American Burn Association, 2006–14.

Although the BRDSS system was initially introduced as a performance improvement project, its use has generated several reportable findings about burn resuscitation. These are summarized in **Table 1**. Most notably, there was a reduction in crystalloid volume, ventilator days, and mortality, with an increase in the frequency of UO within the target range.[42]

SUMMARY

This article reviewed the history of burn resuscitation formulas, and their evolution into paper-based clinical practice guidelines and computerized decision support systems. This experience has highlighted the importance of enhancing situational awareness and team communication during the resuscitation process, a high-risk endeavor in which errors can lead to a host of complications and to increased mortality. Examples of tools that can improve performance include a paper flow sheet that facilitates hand-offs as a casualty is moved through a multitiered aeromedical evacuation chain,[10] and software that prompts (and empowers) nurses and physicians to communicate at key junctures during a difficult resuscitation.[42] Attention to these human factors in the use of critical care technology is as important as the technology itself.

REFERENCES

1. Harkins HN, Lam CR, Romence H. Plasma therapy in severe burns. Surg Gynecol Obstet 1942;75:410–20.

2. Cope O, Moore FD. The redistribution of body water and the fluid therapy of the burned patient. Ann Surg 1947;126:1010–45.
3. Reiss E, Stirman JA, Artz CP, et al. Fluid and electrolyte balance in burns. JAMA 1953;152:1309–13.
4. Shires GT, Cunningham JN, Backer CR, et al. Alterations in cellular membrane function during hemorrhagic shock in primates. Ann Surg 1972;176(3):288–95.
5. Baxter CR, Shires T. Physiological response to crystalloid resuscitation of severe burns. Ann N Y Acad Sci 1968;150(3):874–94.
6. Pruitt BA Jr, Mason AD Jr, Moncrief JA. Hemodynamic changes in the early post-burn patient: the influence of fluid administration and of a vasodilator (hydralazine). J Trauma 1971;11(1):36–46.
7. Greenhalgh DG. Burn resuscitation: the results of the ISBI/ABA survey. Burns 2010;36(2):176–82.
8. Anonymous. Emergency war surgery: third United States revision. Washington, DC: The Borden Institute; 2004.
9. Cancio LC, Mozingo DW, Pruitt BA Jr. The technique of fluid resuscitation for patients with severe thermal injuries. J Crit Illn 1997;12:183–90.
10. Ennis JL, Chung KK, Renz EM, et al. Joint Theater Trauma System implementation of burn resuscitation guidelines improves outcomes in severely burned military casualties. J Trauma 2008;64(2 Suppl):S146–51.
11. Lawrence A, Faraklas I, Watkins H, et al. Colloid administration normalizes resuscitation ratio and ameliorates "fluid creep". J Burn Care Res 2010;31(1):40–7.
12. Anonymous. Precision medicine. Available at: http://www.fda.gov/ScienceResearch/SpecialTopics/PersonalizedMedicine/. Accessed February 29, 2016.
13. Engrav LH, Colescott PL, Kemalyan N, et al. A biopsy of the use of the Baxter formula to resuscitate burns or do we do it like Charlie did it? J Burn Care Rehabil 2000;21(2):91–5.
14. Cancio LC, Chavez S, Alvarado-Ortega M, et al. Predicting increased fluid requirements during the resuscitation of thermally injured patients. J Trauma 2004;56(2):404–13 [discussion: 413–4].
15. Chung KK, Wolf SE, Cancio LC, et al. Resuscitation of severely burned military casualties: fluid begets more fluid. J Trauma 2009;67(2):231–7.
16. Arturson G, Jonsson CE. Transcapillary transport after thermal injury. Scand J Plast Reconstr Surg 1979;13:29–38.
17. Yuan SY, Rigor RR. Pathophysiology and clinical relevance. Chapter 7. In: Yuan SY, Rigor RR, editors. Regulation of endothelial barrier function. San Rafael (CA): Morgan & Claypool Life Sciences; 2010. p. 91–104.
18. Onarheim H, Brofeldt BT, Gunther RA. Markedly increased lymphatic removal of hyaluronan from skin after major thermal injury. Burns 1996;22(3):212–6.
19. Pham TN, Cancio LC, Gibran NS. American Burn Association practice guidelines: burn shock resuscitation. J Burn Care Res 2008;29(1):257–66.
20. Cartotto R, Zhou A. Fluid creep: the pendulum hasn't swung back yet! J Burn Care Res 2010;31(4):551–8.
21. Ivy ME, Atweh NA, Palmer J, et al. Intra-abdominal hypertension and abdominal compartment syndrome in burn patients. J Trauma 2000;49(3):387–91.
22. Sheridan RL, Tompkins RG, McManus WF, et al. Intracompartmental sepsis in burn patients. J Trauma 1994;36(3):301 5.
23. Dulhunty JM, Boots RJ, Rudd MJ, et al. Increased fluid resuscitation can lead to adverse outcomes in major-burn injured patients, but low mortality is achievable. Burns 2008;34(8):1090–7.

24. Zak AL, Harrington DT, Barillo DJ, et al. Acute respiratory failure that complicates the resuscitation of pediatric patients with scald injuries. J Burn Care Rehabil 1999;20(5):391–9.
25. Pruitt BA Jr. Protection from excessive resuscitation: "pushing the pendulum back". J Trauma 2000;49(3):567–8.
26. Eastridge BJ, Jenkins D, Flaherty S, et al. Trauma system development in a theater of war: experiences from Operation Iraqi Freedom and Operation Enduring Freedom. J Trauma 2006;61(6):1366–72.
27. Faraklas I, Lam U, Cochran A, et al. Colloid normalizes resuscitation ratio in pediatric burns. J Burn Care Res 2011;32(1):91–7.
28. Faraklas I, Cochran A, Saffle J. Review of a fluid resuscitation protocol: "fluid creep" is not due to nursing error. J Burn Care Res 2012;33(1):74–83.
29. Jaskille AD, Jeng JC, Sokolich JC, et al. Repetitive ischemia-reperfusion injury: a plausible mechanism for documented clinical burn-depth progression after thermal injury. J Burn Care Res 2007;28(1):13–20.
30. Hoskins SL, Elgjo GI, Lu J, et al. Closed-loop resuscitation of burn shock. J Burn Care Res 2006;27(3):377–85.
31. Bowman RJ, Westenskow DR. A microcomputer-based fluid infusion system for the resuscitation of burn patients. IEEE Trans Biomed Eng 1981;28(6):475–9.
32. Zadeh L. Fuzzy sets. Inform Contr 1965;8:338–53.
33. Hazelzet JA. Can fuzzy logic make things more clear? Crit Care 2009;13(1):116.
34. Ying H, Bonnerup C, Kirschne R, et al. Closed-loop fuzzy control of resuscitation of hemorrhagic shock in sheep. Paper presented at: Engineering in Medicine and Biology. 24th Annual Conference and the Annual Fall Meeting of the Biomedical Engineering Society EMBS/BMES Conference. Houston, TX, October 23–26, 2002.
35. Hedlund A, Zaar B, Groth T, et al. Computer simulation of fluid resuscitation in trauma. I. Description of an extensive pathophysiological model and its first validation. Comput Methods Programs Biomed 1988;27(1):7–21.
36. Arturson G, Groth T, Hedlund A, et al. Computer simulation of fluid resuscitation in trauma. First pragmatic validation in thermal injury. J Burn Care Rehabil 1989; 10(4):292–9.
37. Roa LM, Gomez-Cia T, Cantero A. Analysis of burn injury by digital simulation. Burns 1988;14(3):201–9.
38. Roa L, Gomez-Cia T. A burn patient resuscitation therapy designed by computer simulation (BET). Part 1: simulation studies. Burns 1993;19(4):324–31.
39. Gomez-Cia T, Roa L. A burn patient resuscitation therapy designed by computer simulation (BET). Part 2: initial clinical validation. Burns 1993;19(4):332–8.
40. Ampratwum RT, Bowen BD, Lund T, et al. A model of fluid resuscitation following burn injury: formulation and parameter estimation. Comput Methods Programs Biomed 1995;47(1):1–19.
41. Anonymous. MDDS rule. Available at: http://www.fda.gov/MedicalDevices/Product sandMedicalProcedures/GeneralHospitalDevicesandSupplies/MedicalDeviceData Systems/ucm251897.htm. Accessed February 29, 2016.
42. Salinas J, Chung KK, Mann EA, et al. Computerized decision support system improves fluid resuscitation following severe burns: an original study. Crit Care Med 2011;39(9):2031–8.
43. Cancio LC, Serio-Melvin M, Garcia A, et al. Electronic medical records for burn centers: what do users need? J Burn Care Res 2014;35(2):134–5.

Future Therapies in Burn Resuscitation

Erica I. Hodgman, MD, Madhu Subramanian, MD, Brett D. Arnoldo, MD,
Herb A. Phelan, MD, Steven E. Wolf, MD*

KEYWORDS

- Burns • Fluid resuscitation • Monitoring • Fluid creep

KEY POINTS

- Hourly urine output remains the gold standard to guide resuscitation.
- Early administration of colloids, including albumin and/or fresh frozen plasma should be considered.
- Management of the hypermetabolic state, including nutritional support and pharmacologic agents, should be initiated as early as possible.
- Use of computer-based burn size calculators and decision support algorithms may improve outcomes.

INTRODUCTION

In the 1940s, 2 major fires, the Cocoanut Grove Fire and the Texas City disaster, ushered in the modern era of burn care.[1] The clinical observations following these disasters prompted new lines of scientific inquiry, leading researchers to demonstrate that severe burns result not only in the loss of the intrinsic barrier function of the skin but also severe systemic inflammation. Cope and Moore[2,3] established the relationship between burn size and fluid loss and the phenomenon of capillary leak, which caused significant edema even in uninjured areas. Cuthbertson and colleagues[4] described the ebb and flow periods following significant trauma, which would prove particularly relevant to burns. The clinical relevance of these 2 phases was underscored by Reiss and colleagues[5] in 1953, when they proposed an algorithm that used a large volume of fluid (including colloid) in the first 8 hours, followed by a tapering of the infusion rate. This would eventually lead to the establishment of the Parkland Burn Formula by Baxter and Shires[6] in 1968, and the Brooke Formula by Drs Pruitt, Mason, and Moncrief.[5]

The 1970s brought a clearer picture of the metabolic derangements that plague burn patients.[7] Perhaps most strikingly, Long and colleagues[8] demonstrated that

External Funding: Gracious support has been provided by the Pettis family through Sons of the Flag.

Division of Burns, Trauma, and Critical Care, Department of Surgery, University of Texas–Southwestern Medical Center, 5323 Harry Hines Boulevard, Dallas, TX 75390-9158, USA
* Corresponding author.
E-mail address: steven.wolf@utsouthwestern.edu

Crit Care Clin 32 (2016) 611–619
http://dx.doi.org/10.1016/j.ccc.2016.06.009
0749-0704/16/© 2016 Elsevier Inc. All rights reserved.

patients with severe burns have a drastic increase in energy expenditure over resting metabolic rate and urinary nitrogen excretion rates far exceeding even that of patients with severe musculoskeletal trauma. This hypermetabolism would eventually be linked to muscle atrophy, impaired rehabilitation, and increased risk of sepsis and mortality.[9] These findings pushed clinicians toward early enteral feeding and beta blockade in an effort to mitigate the ill effects of a prolonged hypermetabolic state.[7,10–12]

The 1980s through the 2000s have witnessed a transition to a more mechanistic understanding of these physiologic changes, with increasing studies into the role of inflammatory cytokines and alterations in genetic expression.[13,14] There has also been an increasing focus on the role of technology in the initial management of burn patients, with use of computerized resuscitation algorithms and sophisticated invasive and noninvasive monitoring. As is often the case with research, there more questions than answers left in the search for the optimal approach to the initial resuscitation of the burned patient. Advances are expected in the near future that will result in meaningful improvements in mortality, morbidity, and functional outcomes.

RESUSCITATIVE FLUIDS

Without resuscitation, the rapid massive shifts in both fluid volume and sodium mass that follow a significant burn result in cardiovascular collapse and death.[2,3,5] Traditionally, the treatment of choice has been a balanced salt solution to replete intravascular volume and sodium without an excess of chloride to worsen the metabolic acidosis that is usually present.[6,15] Indeed, lactated Ringer solution is the resuscitation fluid of choice of 91% of burn care providers.[16] Although some argue for the use of hypertonic solutions to more efficiently replete sodium stores, the risk of subsequent severe hypernatremia and evidence suggesting an increased incidence of acute renal failure has prevented its widespread adoption.[17,18]

The use of colloids, however, remains far more intriguing and controversial. Increased capillary permeability is most pronounced and prolonged in burned tissues but also occurs to a lesser degree and shorter duration in noninjured tissue.[3,19] Clinicians, therefore, surmised that administration of large molecular weight proteins before restoration of capillary integrity increases neither intravascular oncotic pressure nor volume and could result in prolonged edema. Several meta-analyses demonstrated worse outcomes among critically ill patients resuscitated with albumin versus crystalloid alone; however, the applicability of these analyses, which were based on studies with heterogeneous populations and often excluded burn patients, to a burn population are limited.[20,21] In contrast, animal models of severe burn suggest that colloid administration actually decreases fluid translocation in nonburned tissues and, indeed, randomized controlled trials among burn patients have found that routine use of albumin during the initial resuscitation period led to decreased fluid administration.[19,22,23] Although some of these studies also reported an increased risk of mortality or other complications associated with early albumin administration, they have limitations that weaken the strength of these associations and newer high quality data are not available.[22] Moreover, surveys suggest that albumin is more frequently used as a rescue therapy rather than as a standard component of the resuscitation formula.[16,18] Thus, the lack of more conclusive evidence in support of colloid therapy may be due in part because patients who are given albumin in response to resuscitation failure are already experiencing the deleterious effects of a massive volume of crystalloid.

Although albumin is the most commonly used colloid today, its commercial availability is a relatively recent development.[16] In fact, other products, including plasma and whole blood, were the colloids used during the derivation of most commonly cited resuscitation protocols.[19] The routine use of blood products was abandoned due to the relative scarcity of resources along with concerns about the risk of infection and transfusion-associated acute lung injury.[18] However, newer evidence suggests fresh frozen plasma (FFP), which contains proinflammatory and anti-inflammatory, and pro-coagulant and anticoagulant, factors, may exert additional beneficial effects not seen following administration of albumin.[24] In the only recent trial using FFP, O'Mara and colleagues[25] found that subjects treated with FFP received less volume overall, had lower mean peak airway and intra-abdominal pressures, and were more likely to correct their base deficit. Unfortunately, it remains unclear whether these outcomes were the result of increased intravascular oncotic pressure alone, or were related to the immunomodulatory effects of FFP.[24] Although the presence of coagulopathy following a burn remains controversial, it seems logical that preferential use of FFP as a colloid during resuscitation would be of benefit to a patient with evidence of coagulopathy.[26,27]

Other colloids will likely remain infrequently used, due in large part to their unfavorable side-effect profiles. A systematic review of the evidence suggests an increased risk of coagulopathy, acute kidney injury, prolonged refractory pruritus, and even death following administration of hydroxyethyl starch solutions.[28,29] Gelatin solutions have similarly been associated with a 2-fold increased risk of acute renal failure.[28]

RESUSCITATION VOLUMES

Fluid resuscitation following a severe burn remains a delicate goal. Under-resuscitation leads to hypoperfusion, end-organ damage, and death; whereas over-resuscitation leads to abdominal and extremity compartment syndromes, pulmonary edema, and death. Thus, the optimal resuscitation results in administration of neither too little nor too much fluid (the Goldilocks principle).[30,31] The Parkland Formula and the modified Brooke Formula remain the most commonly used methods to estimate initial fluid infusion rates.[6,16,18] Although it has long been known that certain subsets of patients, specifically those with electrical injuries or electrical burns, require fluid in excess of predicted volumes, the phenomenon of fluid creep is increasingly being recognized as a problem.[15,32] The cause of fluid creep is likely multifactorial, stemming from the proliferation of new goals used in goal-directed therapy (eg, base deficit, lactate, cardiac index and/or output, and surrogate markers, such as stroke volume variation), increased opioid utilization, increased fluid administration by emergency medical transport teams, and the reduced utilization of colloids.[19,32,33]

One very promising avenue of research is the use of computerized decision-support tools, like that developed at the US Army Institute of Surgical Research that was shown to decrease the volume of crystalloid infused and, subsequently the incidence of abdominal compartment syndrome.[34] In comparison, other groups who used a more conservative but not computerized protocol showed a less dramatic reduction in average fluid volumes.[35,36] This is likely because it is cognitively easier to turn the fluid rate up than it is to turn it down. Thus, computer algorithms provide recommendations that can actually result in improved outcomes. As integration of electronic medical records systems into the intensive care unit continues to improve, it is likely that computerized decision support aid will become more commonplace.

Another factor that likely contributes to over-resuscitation is an inaccurate assessment of burn size. The rule of nines has been popularized for several decades, yet burn centers frequently encounter patients whose reported burn size far exceed their actual injury burden and have, consequently, received a significant excess of crystalloid. Clinicians are working toward a computer-assisted or, perhaps, even a smartphone application-based, method to provide an objective, rather than subjective, assessment of burn size and, perhaps, burn depth.[37–40] There has not yet been a trial that demonstrates improved accuracy of burn size estimation nor the subsequent fluid rate calculations provided by these applications.

High-dose ascorbic acid is the only pharmacologic agent currently under trial that may have efficacy in reducing resuscitation volumes.[41] Although many studies have evaluated its efficacy, it still has not gained traction, perhaps due to a perceived risk of osmotic diuresis and renal failure or the association with pseudohyperglycemia, which can further muddy the picture of a critically ill patient.[41,42]

By debulking the devitalized, inflammatory burned tissue, early excision of burn wounds may also diminish the duration or degree of capillary leak in nonburned tissues.[43] Unfortunately, studies directly evaluating the effect of early excision on resuscitation volumes (after correcting for blood loss) have not yet been performed.

APPROACHES TO MONITORING

As technology marches forward, the number of potential resuscitation endpoints continues to proliferate. Both Drs Baxter and Shires,[6] and Pruitt[15] envisioned their formulae as a starting point for the titration fluid infusion rates to maintain a urinary output of 0.5 to 1.0 mL/kg/h, and most clinicians report urinary output remains their primary resuscitation endpoint.[6,15,16] Modalities now used in the modern intensive care unit include transthoracic and/or transesophageal echocardiography, central venous pressure, measures of cardiac preload or fluid responsiveness (ie, percent stroke volume variation, intrathoracic blood volume index [ITBVI] or pulmonary arterial wedge pressure, cardiac index), measures of oxygen delivery and/or consumption (eg, central venous oxygen saturation [$ScvO_2$]), serum markers (eg, base deficit, lactate), and measures of cellular metabolism (eg, gastric tonometry, confocal laser-scanning microscopy, near-infrared spectroscopy, sidestream dark-field video microscopy).[44–47] These approaches to monitoring are useful only if they provide real-time data to guide a clinician's actions in a meaningful way. For example, in a patient with a large burn, the most important monitor is perhaps the bladder pressure monitor because a patient who approaches an Ivy index of 250 cc/kg is at significant risk of intra-abdominal hypertension or abdominal compartment syndrome and may benefit from an alteration of resuscitation strategy (eg, incorporation of more colloids or perhaps even hypertonic solutions).[48]

The major pitfall of monitoring more parameters is that clinicians can begin to chase too many goals, and many of these new measures have not been validated as a resuscitative endpoint in a burn patient population. This is thought to be among the myriad causes of the phenomenon of fluid creep, as discussed previously.[32] A small randomized controlled trial evaluating the use of ITBVI to guide fluid resuscitation demonstrated that experimental patients received significantly more fluid than those who were resuscitated based on hourly urine output alone, and there were no improvements in mortality, overall incidence of multisystem organ failure, or hospital length of stay.[49] A separate prospective trial of an algorithm that incorporated both lactate and ITBVI values also found no relationship between urinary output and other markers of resuscitation, and further reported that it was possible to have normalization of lactate and cardiac index even in the face of a low ITBVI.[50] Similarly, Papp and colleagues[51] found that patients who received nearly double the volume predicted by the Parkland Formula and had an adequate hourly urinary output, nevertheless had evidence of hypovolemia on transesophageal echo. Further illustration is provided by a historical case-control series that evaluated the use of a permissive hypovolemia algorithm, and found no increase in adverse outcomes.[52]

It is likely that hourly urinary output will remain the ultimate marker of adequate resuscitation and end-organ perfusion because it requires no specialized equipment, carries little risk apart from that of catheter-related urinary tract infection, and is easy to interpret. Serial calculations of a patient's KMAC ratio, simply the ratio of hourly rate of fluids administration (mL/kg/%TBSA/h) to the hourly urine output (mL/kg), may provide a more nuanced way to monitor the progress of their resuscitation.[53] Use of more advanced monitoring systems may be of benefit for patients who have preinjury comorbidities that complicate the bedside assessment of volume status, such as those with chronic kidney disease or congestive heart failure, or for those who are failing their fluid resuscitation (eg, receiving volumes far in excess of that predicted by the Parkland Formula).

THE HYPERMETABOLIC STATE

Though the stigmata of the hypermetabolic state that follows a severe burn have been apparent for decades, researchers have only recently begun to more fully appreciate the detrimental sequelae of the flow phase of burn recovery.[7,11] The underlying mechanisms by which this massive metabolic, hormonal, and inflammatory dysregulation occur are still being actively investigated. Xiao and colleagues[14] provided a 30,000-foot view of the magnitude of the genomic storm that occurs within 24 hours of injury, with alteration in expression of more than 5000 genes that, among burn patients, persists up to 90 days or longer. Further research is needed to determine whether this information can be translated to the bedside by using alterations in gene expression patterns to identify patients at risk for complications, such as resuscitative failure, multisystem organ failure, and infection.

Nutritional support, the simplest intervention available to any clinician, plays a vital role in the management of any burn patient. Early investigations using both animal models and burn patients demonstrated the ability of early enteral nutrition to mitigate burn-induced hypercatabolism.[12] The effects of nutritional support not only include improved muscle mass maintenance but also modulation of stress hormone levels, improved gut mucosal integrity, improved wound healing, decreased risk of Curling ulcer formation, and a shorter intensive care unit length of stay.[12,54–56] Early enteral nutrition, including a protein intake of 1.5 to 2 g/kg/d has been and will continue to be a mainstay of burn resuscitation therapy.[9] Supplementation with amino acids, such as glutamine, arginine, and leucine, may also be of some benefit, although more data are needed.[9]

Another weapon in the battle against the hypermetabolic response is early excision and grafting for patients with a large injury burden.[57,58] Studies into the effects of early excision have shown improvements in mortality, decreased exudative protein loss, and lower risk of burn wound infection, and an expected increased rate of blood product utilization, suggesting that early excision is a resource-intensive but lifesaving intervention.[59,60] These effects may be due in part to a substantial decrease in the circulating levels of inflammatory cytokines, including interleukin (IL)-6, IL-8, C3 complement, and tumor necrosis factor-α.[43] The benefits of early excision will likely be further compounded by advances in wound management. There are several new products currently being investigated that, unlike current allograft and xenograft products, allow immediate permanent wound coverage, eliminate the creation of donor site (and the subsequent physiologic stress of additional wound burden to heal), and limit the number of operations to achieve wound closure.[61]

There are several proven pharmacologic approaches to attenuate the hypermetabolic flow phase of a burn. Adrenergic blockade (most commonly with propranolol) has favorable effects on heart rate, resting energy expenditure, oxygen consumption, and net muscle-protein balance.[7,11] Insulin therapy promotes maintenance of muscle mass and improved donor site healing, without increasing hepatic triglyceride synthesis.[62,63] Oxandrolone, a synthetic androgen, has been shown to increase both muscle protein synthesis and muscle strength, as well as improve bone mineral content.[10,64] Recombinant human growth hormone (rHGH) remains more controversial. Although it has beneficial effects on both serum markers of inflammation and long-term clinical outcomes, such as wound healing, scar formation, and bone and mineral density, there are concerns that rHGH therapy may increase the risk of mortality among critically ill, nonburn, adult patients.[65,66]

SUMMARY

The ideal burn resuscitation limits the volume of fluid infused; tempers the negative effects of the postburn hypermetabolic, hyperinflammatory state; and promotes rapid wound healing to allow patients to begin the rehabilitation phase of their care as early as possible. The authors believe that the burn resuscitation of the future is likely to look very much like the resuscitation of the 1970s or 1980s, modernized with the integration of decision-support algorithms into the electronic medical record system. Patients will be resuscitated with both crystalloid and colloid, perhaps in the form of FFP or other blood products, titrated with the assistance of a computerized algorithm to maintain an hourly urine output between 0.5 and 1.0 cc/kg. Enteral nutrition and early excision will remain mainstays of therapy, and the routine addition of beta blockade and anabolic or anticatabolic agents will act synergistically to prevent lean muscle mass loss. The authors hope that rapid genomic analysis will be used to further tailor the selection of adjunct therapies for patients. Additionally, novel wound products that allow for permanent initial closure of burn wounds without the creation of a donor site will eliminate the second hit that patients currently take during autologous skin grafting.

REFERENCES

1. Pruitt BA Jr, Wolf SE. An historical perspective on advances in burn care over the past 100 years. Clin Plast Surg 2009;36:527–45.
2. Cope O, Moore FD. The redistribution of body water and the fluid therapy of the burned patient. Ann Surg 1947;126:1010–45.
3. Cope O, Moore FD. A study of capillary permeability in experimental burns and burn shock using radioactive dyes in blood and lymph. J Clin Invest 1944; 23(2):241–57.
4. Cuthbertson DP, Angeles Valero Zanuy MA, León Sanz ML. Post-shock metabolic response. 1942. Nutr Hosp 2001;16(5):176–82.
5. Pruitt BA Jr. Fluid and electrolyte replacement in the burned patient. Surg Clin North Am 1978;58:1291–312.
6. Baxter CR, Shires T. Physiological response to crystalloid resuscitation of severe burns. Ann N Y Acad Sci 1968;150:874–94.
7. Wilmore DW, Long JM, Mason AD Jr, et al. Catecholamines: mediator of the hypermetabolic response to thermal injury. Ann Surg 1974;180:653–69.
8. Long CL, Schaffel N, Geiger JW, et al. Metabolic response to injury and illness: estimation of energy and protein needs for indirect calorimetry and nitrogen balance. JPEN J Parenter Enteral Nutr 1979;3(6):452–6.

9. Chang DW, DeSanti L, Demling RH. Anticatabolic and anabolic strategies in critical illness: a review of current treatment modalities. Shock 1998;10:155–60.

10. Wolf SE, Thomas SJ, Dasu MR, et al. Improved net protein balance, lean mass, and gene expression changes with oxandrolone treatment in the severely burned. Ann Surg 2003;237(6):801–10.

11. Herndon DN, Hart DW, Wolf SE, et al. Reversal of catabolism by beta-blockade after severe burns. N Engl J Med 2001;345:1223–9.

12. Mochizuki H, Trocki O, Dominioni L, et al. Mechanism of prevention of postburn hypermetabolism and catabolism by early enteral feeding. Ann Surg 1984;200: 297–310.

13. Finnerty CC, Ju H, Spratt H, et al. Proteomics improves the prediction of burns mortality: results from regression spline modeling. Clin Transl Sci 2012;5:243–9.

14. Xiao W, Mindrinos MN, Seok J, et al. A genomic storm in critically injured humans. J Exp Med 2011;208(13):2581–90.

15. Pruitt BA Jr. Advances in fluid therapy and the early care of the burn patient. World J Surg 1978;2:139–50.

16. Greenhalgh DG. Burn resuscitation: the results of the ISBI/ABA survey. Burns 2010;36:176–82.

17. Monafo WW. The treatment of burn shock by the intravenous and oral administration of hypertonic lactated saline solution. J Trauma 1970;10:575–86.

18. Pham TN, Cancio LC, Gibran NS, et al. American Burn Association practice guidelines burn shock resuscitation. J Burn Care Res 2008;29:257–66.

19. Cartotto R, Callum J. A review of the use of human albumin in burn patients. J Burn Care Res 2012;33:702–17.

20. Roberts I, Blackhall K, Alderson P, et al. Human albumin solution for resuscitation and volume expansion in critically ill patients. Cochrane Database Syst Rev 2011;(11):CD001208.

21. Perel P, Roberts I. Colloids versus crystalloids for fluid resuscitation in critically ill patients. Cochrane Database Syst Rev 2013;(2):CD000567.

22. Goodwin CW, Dorothy J, Lam V, et al. Randomized trial of efficacy of crystalloid and colloid resuscitation on hemodynamic response and lung water following thermal injury. Ann Surg 1983;197:520–31.

23. Demling RH, Kramer G, Harms B. Role of thermal injury-induced hypoproteinemia on fluid flux and protein permeability in burned and nonburned tissue. Surgery 1984;95:136–44.

24. Vamvakas EC, Blajchman MA. Transfusion-related immunomodulation (TRIM): an update. Blood Rev 2007;21:327–48.

25. O'Mara MS, Slater H, Goldfarb IW. A prospective, randomized evaluation of intra-abdominal pressures with crystalloid and colloid resuscitation in burn patients. J Trauma 2005;58(5):1011–8.

26. Sherren PB, Hussey J, Martin R, et al. Acute burn induced coagulopathy. Burns 2013;39(6):1157–61.

27. Van Haren RM, Thorson CM, Valle EJ, et al. Hypercoagulability after burn injury. J Trauma 2013;75(1):37–43.

28. Groeneveld AB, Navickis RJ, Wilkes MM. Update on the comparative safety of colloids: a systematic review of clinical studies. Ann Surg 2011;253:470–83.

29. Béchir M, Puhan MA, Neff SB, et al. Early fluid resuscitation with hyperoncotic hydroxyethyl starch 200/0.5 (10%) in severe burn injury. Crit Care 2010;14(3):R123.

30. Ivy ME, Atweh NA, Palmer J, et al. Intra-abdominal hypertension and abdominal compartment syndrome in burn patients. J Trauma 2000;49:387–91.

31. Latenser BA. Critical care of the burn patient: the first 48 hours. Crit Care Med 2009;37:2819–26.
32. Saffle JI. The phenomenon of "fluid creep" in acute burn resuscitation. J Burn Care Res 2007;28:382–95.
33. Sullivan SR, Friedrich JB, Engrav LH, et al. "Opioid creep" is real and may be the cause of "fluid creep". Burns 2004;30:583–90.
34. Salinas J, Chung KK, Mann EA, et al. Computerized decision support system improves fluid resuscitation following severe burns: an original study. Crit Care Med 2011;39:2031–8.
35. Mitchell KB, Khalil E, Brennan A, et al. New management strategy for fluid resuscitation: quantifying volume in the first 48 hours after burn injury. J Burn Care Res 2013;34:196–202.
36. Faraklas I, Cochran A, Saffle J. Review of a fluid resuscitation protocol: "Fluid creep" is not due to nursing error. J Burn Care Res 2012;33:74–83.
37. Kamolz LP, Wurzer P, Giretzlehner M, et al. Burn surface area calculation instead of burn size estimation: our opinion. Burns 2014;40:1813–4.
38. Kamolz LP, Parvizi D, Giretzlehner M, et al. Burn surface area calculation: what do we need in future. Burns 2014;40:171–2.
39. Giretzlehner M, Dirnberger J, Owen R, et al. The determination of total burn surface area: how much difference? Burns 2013;39:1107–13.
40. Morris R, Javed M, Bodger O, et al. A comparison of two smartphone applications and the validation of smartphone applications as tools for fluid calculation for burns resuscitation. Burns 2014;40:826–34.
41. Kahn SA, Beers RJ, Lentz CW. Resuscitation after severe burn injury using high-dose ascorbic acid: a retrospective review. J Burn Care Res 2011;32:110–7.
42. Kahn SA, Lentz CW. Fictitious hyperglycemia: point-of-care glucose measurement is inaccurate during high-dose vitamin C infusion for burn shock resuscitation. J Burn Care Res 2015;36:e67–71.
43. Barret JP, Herndon DN. Modulation of inflammatory and catabolic responses in severely burned children by early burn wound excision in the first 24 hours. Arch Surg 2003;138(2):127–32.
44. Paratz JD, Stockton K, Paratz ED, et al. Burn resuscitation-hourly urine output versus alternative endpoints: a systematic review. Shock 2014;42:295–306.
45. Foldi V, Csontos C, Bogar L, et al. Effects of fluid resuscitation methods on burn trauma-induced oxidative stress. J Burn Care Res 2009;30:957–66.
46. Altintas MA, Altintas AA, Guggenheim M, et al. Insight in microcirculation and histomorphology during burn shock treatment using in vivo confocal-laser-scanning microscopy. J Crit Care 2010;25:173.e1-7.
47. Dries DJ, Waxman K. Adequate resuscitation of burn patients may not be measured by urine output and vital signs. Crit Care Med 1991;19(3):327–9.
48. Cancio LC. Initial assessment and fluid resuscitation of burn patients. Surg Clin North Am 2014;94:741–54.
49. Foldi V, Lantos J, Bogar L, et al. Effects of fluid resuscitation methods on the pro- and anti-inflammatory cytokines and expression of adhesion molecules after burn injury. J Burn Care Res 2010;31:480–91.
50. Sanchez M, García-de-Lorenzo A, Herrero E, et al. A protocol for resuscitation of severe burn patients guided by transpulmonary thermodilution and lactate levels: a 3-year prospective cohort study. Crit Care 2013;17:R176.
51. Papp A, Uusaro A, Parviainen I, et al. Mycoardial function and haemodynamics in extensive burn trauma: evaluation by clinical signs, invasive monitoring,

echocardiography, and cytokine concentrations. A prospective clinical study. Acta Anaesthesiol Scand 2003;47(10):1257–63.

52. Arlati S, Storti E, Pradella V, et al. Decreased fluid volume to reduce organ damage: a new approach to burn shock resuscitation? A preliminary study. Resuscitation 2007;72:371–8.

53. Kelly JF, McLaughlin DF, Oppenheimer JH, et al. A novel means to classify response to resuscitation in the severely burned: derivation of the KMAC value. Burns 2013;39:1060–6.

54. Mosier MJ, Pham TN, Klein MB, et al. Early enteral nutrition in burns: compliance with guidelines and associated outcomes in a multicenter study. J Burn Care Res 2011;32:104–9.

55. Peng YZ, Yuan ZQ, Xiao GX. Effects of early enteral feeding on the prevention of enterogenic infection in severely burned patients. Burns 2001;27:145–9.

56. Xiao SC. Prevention and treatment of gastrointestinal dysfunction following severe burns: a summary of recent 30-year clinical experience. World J Gastroenterol 2008;14:3231.

57. Janzekovic Z. A new concept in the early excision and immediate grafting of burns. J Trauma 1970;10:1103–8.

58. Herndon DN, Barrow RE, Rutan RL, et al. A comparison of conservative versus early excision. Ann Surg 1989;209(5):547–52.

59. Ong YS, Samuel M, Song C. Meta-analysis of early excision of burns. Burns 2006; 32:145–50.

60. Hart DW, Wolf SE, Chinkes DL, et al. Effects of early excision and aggressive enteral feeding on hypermetabolism, catabolism, and sepsis after severe burn. J Trauma 2003;54(4):755–61.

61. Rowan MP, Cancio LC, Elster EA, et al. Burn wound healing and treatment: review and advancements. Crit Care 2015;19:243.

62. Thomas SJ, Morimoto K, Herndon DN, et al. The effect of prolonged euglycemic hyperinsulinemia on lean body mass after severe burn. Surgery 2002;132:341–7.

63. Herndon DN, Tompkins RG. Support of the metabolic response to burn injury. Lancet 2004;363:1895–902.

64. Wolf SE, Edelman LS, Kemalyan N, et al. Effects of oxandrolone on outcome measures in the severely burned: a multicenter prospective randomized double-blind trial. J Burn Care Res 2006;27(2):131–9.

65. Williams FN, Jeschke MG, Chinkes DL, et al. Modulation of the hypermetabolic response to trauma: temperature, nutrition, and drugs. J Am Coll Surg 2009; 208:489–502.

66. Klein GL, Wolf SE, Langman CB, et al. Effect of therapy with recombinant human growth hormone on insulin-like growth factor system components and serum levels of biochemical markers of bone formation in children after severe burn injury. J Clin Endocrinol Metab 1998;83(1):21–4.

Index

Note: Page numbers of article titles are in **boldface** type.

A

Albumin
   in acute burn resuscitation, 514–515
Antioxidant(s)
   in burn resuscitation, 540–541
Arterial waveform pulse analysis
   in hemodynamic monitoring of end points of burn resuscitation, 528–529
Ascorbic acid
   high-dose
      in fluid creep management, 595
Austere environment
   burn resuscitation in, **561–565** (*See also* Burn resuscitation, in austere environment)

B

Base deficit
   in monitoring end points of burn resuscitation, 530–531
Burn(s)
   acute
      fluid resuscitation for
         colloids in, **507–523** (*See also* Colloid(s), in acute burn resuscitation)
Burn edema
   hypovolemia and, 492–496
Burn injury(ies)
   aggressive fluid resuscitation after, **491–505**
   in austere environment, **561–565**
      evaluation overview, 562–563
      introduction, 561–562
      long-term recommendations for, 564
      outcomes of, 564
      pharmacologic agents for, 563–564
   in children (*See* Children, burn injuries in)
   increased capillary permeability due to, 540
   mediators of
      inflammatory cytokines as, 498–501
   multiorgan dysfunction after, 496–498
   pathophysiology of, 540
Burn resuscitation
   for acute burns
      colloids in, **507–523** (*See also* Colloid(s), in acute burn resuscitation)
   antioxidant therapy in, 540–541
   in austere environment, **561–565**

Crit Care Clin 32 (2016) 621–627
http://dx.doi.org/10.1016/S0749-0704(16)30075-6
0749-0704/16/$ – see front matter

UNITED STATES POSTAL SERVICE® Statement of Ownership, Management, and Circulation
(All Periodicals Publications Except Requester Publications)

1. Publication Title	2. Publication Number	3. Filing Date
CRITICAL CARE CLINICS	000 – 708	9/18/2015

4. Issue Frequency	5. Number of Issues Published Annually	6. Annual Subscription Price
JAN, APR, JUL, OCT	4	$199.00

7. Complete Mailing Address of Known Office of Publication (Not printer) (Street, city, county, state, and ZIP+4®)

ELSEVIER INC.
360 PARK AVENUE SOUTH
NEW YORK, NY 10010-1710

Contact Person
STEPHEN R. BUSHING

Telephone (Include area code)
2 t 5-239-3688

8. Complete Mailing Address of Headquarters or General Business Office of Publisher (Not printer)

ELSEVIER INC.
360 PARK AVENUE SOUTH
NEW YORK, NY 10010-1710

9. Full Names and Complete Mailing Addresses of Publisher, Editor, and Managing Editor (Do not leave blank)

Publisher (Name and complete mailing address)

ADRIANNE BRIGIDO, ELSEVIER INC.
1600 JOHN F KENNEDY BLVD. SUITE 1800
PHILADELPHIA, PA 19103-2899

Editor (Name and complete mailing address)

KATIE PFAFF, ELSEVIER INC.
1600 JOHN F KENNEDY BLVD. SUITE 1800
PHILADELPHIA, PA 19103-2899

Managing Editor (Name and complete mailing address)

PATRICK MANLEY, ELSEVIER INC.
1600 JOHN F KENNEDY BLVD. SUITE 1800
PHILADELPHIA, PA 19103-2899

10. Owner (Do not leave blank. If the publication is owned by a corporation, give the name and address of the corporation immediately followed by the names and addresses of all stockholders owning or holding 1 percent or more of the total amount of stock. If not owned by a corporation, give the names and addresses of the individual owners. If owned by a partnership or other unincorporated firm, give its name and address as well as those of each individual owner. If the publication is published by a nonprofit organization, give its name and address.)

Full Name	Complete Mailing Address
WHOLLY OWNED SUBSIDIARY OF REED/ELSEVIER, US HOLDINGS	1600 JOHN F KENNEDY BLVD. SUITE 1800 PHILADELPHIA, PA 19103-2899

11. Known Bondholders, Mortgagees, and Other Security Holders Owning or Holding 1 Percent or More of Total Amount of Bonds, Mortgages, or Other Securities. If none, check box ► ☐ None

Full Name	Complete Mailing Address
N/A	

12. Tax Status (For completion by nonprofit organizations authorized to mail at nonprofit rates) (Check one)
The purpose, function, and nonprofit status of this organization and the exempt status for federal income tax purposes:
☒ Has Not Changed During Preceding 12 Months
☐ Has Changed During Preceding 12 Months (Publisher must submit explanation of change with this statement)

13. Publication Title	14. Issue Date for Circulation Data Below
CRITICAL CARE CLINICS	JULY 2016

15. Extent and Nature of Circulation			Average No. Copies Each Issue During Preceding 12 Months	No. Copies of Single Issue Published Nearest to Filing Date
a. Total Number of Copies (Net press run)			545	727
b. Paid Circulation (By Mail and Outside the Mail)	(1)	Mailed Outside-County Paid Subscriptions Stated on PS Form 3541 (Include paid distribution above nominal rate, advertiser's proof copies, and exchange copies)	233	301
	(2)	Mailed In-County Paid Subscriptions Stated on PS Form 3541 (Include paid distribution above nominal rate, advertiser's proof copies, and exchange copies)	0	0
	(3)	Paid Distribution Outside the Mails Including Sales Through Dealers and Carriers, Street Vendors, Counter Sales, and Other Paid Distribution Outside USPS®	111	140
	(4)	Paid Distribution by Other Classes of Mail Through the USPS (e.g., First-Class Mail®)	0	0
c. Total Paid Distribution (Sum of 15b (1), (2), (3), and (4))		►	344	441
d. Free or Nominal Rate Distribution (By Mail and Outside the Mail)	(1)	Free or Nominal Rate Outside-County Copies included on PS Form 3541	53	71
	(2)	Free or Nominal Rate In-County Copies Included on PS Form 3541	0	0
	(3)	Free or Nominal Rate Copies Mailed at Other Classes Through the USPS (e.g. First-Class Mail)	0	0
	(4)	Free or Nominal Rate Distribution Outside the Mail (Carriers or other means)	0	0
e. Total Free or Nominal Rate Distribution (Sum of 15d (1), (2), (3) and (4))		►	53	71
f. Total Distribution (Sum of 15c and 15e)		►	397	512
g. Copies not Distributed (See Instructions to Publishers #4 (page #3))		►	148	215
h. Total (Sum of 15f and g)		►	545	727
i. Percent Paid (15c divided by 15f times 100)		►	87%	86%

* If you are claiming electronic copies, go to line 16 on page 3. If you are not claiming electronic copies, skip to line 17 on page 3.

16. Electronic Copy Circulation	Average No. Copies Each Issue During Preceding 12 Months	No. Copies of Single Issue Published Nearest to Filing Date
a. Paid Electronic Copies ►		
b. Total Paid Print Copies (Line 15c) + Paid Electronic Copies (Line 16a) ►	344	441
c. Total Print Distribution (Line 15f) + Paid Electronic Copies (Line 16a) ►	397	512
d. Percent Paid (Both Print & Electronic Copies) (16b divided by 16c × 100) ►	87%	86%

☒ I certify that 50% of all my distributed copies (electronic and print) are paid above a nominal price.

17. Publication of Statement of Ownership
☒ If the publication is a general publication, publication of this statement is required. Will be printed
in the OCTOBER 2016 issue of this publication.

☐ Publication not required.

18. Signature and Title of Editor, Publisher, Business Manager, or Owner

STEPHEN R. BUSHING - INVENTORY DISTRIBUTION CONTROL MANAGER

Date 9/18/2016

I certify that all information furnished on this form is true and complete. I understand that anyone who furnishes false or misleading information on this form or who omits material or information requested on the form may be subject to criminal sanctions (including fines and imprisonment) and/or civil sanctions (including civil penalties).

PS Form 3526, July 2014 (Page 3 of 4)

PRIVACY NOTICE: See our privacy policy on www.usps.com

PS Form 3526, July 2014 (Page 1 of 4 (see instructions page 4)) PSN: 7530-01-000-9931 PRIVACY NOTICE: See our privacy policy on www.usps.com.

Moving?

Make sure your subscription moves with you!

To notify us of your new address, find your **Clinics Account Number** (located on your mailing label above your name), and contact customer service at:

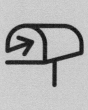

Email: journalscustomerservice-usa@elsevier.com

800-654-2452 (subscribers in the U.S. & Canada)
314-447-8871 (subscribers outside of the U.S. & Canada)

Fax number: 314-447-8029

Elsevier Health Sciences Division
Subscription Customer Service
3251 Riverport Lane
Maryland Heights, MO 63043

*To ensure uninterrupted delivery of your subscription, please notify us at least 4 weeks in advance of move.

ELSEVIER

Printed and bound by CPI Group (UK) Ltd, Croydon, CR0 4YY

03/10/2024

01040400-0009